DIABETES EXPLAINED

DIABETES EXPLAINED

DR ARNOLD BLOOM

THIRD EDITION

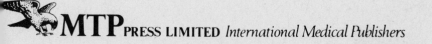 **MTP**PRESS LIMITED *International Medical Publishers*

Published by

MTP PRESS LIMITED

Falcon House
Lancaster, England

Copyright © 1978 Dr Arnold Bloom

ISBN: 0 85200 240 8

First edition 1971
Second edition 1975
Third edition 1978

Photoset, printed and bound
in Great Britain by
REDWOOD BURN LIMITED
Trowbridge & Esher

CONTENTS

PREFACE TO THIRD EDITION

Diabetes is a very common disorder that can occur at any age. It is compatible with a full and healthy life but this demands self discipline and knowledge. It is unreasonable to expect anyone to accept restrictions without understanding the reasons for them.

This book sets out to explain just what diabetes is and how it can be managed successfully. It is intended to help those who have developed diabetes and to interest others who want to understand the implications of this common disorder. Experience with the earlier editions has shown the book to be of value not only to those with diabetes but also to nurses who have to look after diabetic patients. In this third edition opportunity has been taken to bring the book up to date and to expand some sections of practical importance.

It is my earnest hope that this book will continue to prove instructive to those who have diabetes and to those who help to look after them.

ARNOLD BLOOM

London, 1978

SI UNITS

An internationally agreed version of the metric system (Système International) is now being used by many British hospitals. This means that blood sugars are often expressed as mmol/litre instead of mg/dl as used in the text of this book. For example;

$$18 \text{ mg/dl} = 1 \text{ mmol/l}$$
$$90 \text{ mg/dl} = 5 \text{ mmol/l}$$
$$180 \text{ mg/dl} = 10 \text{ mmol/dl}$$

In nutrition, calorie intake is referred to as energy intake. A low calorie diet is referred to as a controlled energy diet and the energy value of food is being expressed as joules instead of calories.

$$1 \text{ calorie} = 4 \cdot 2 \text{ kilojoules (kJ)}$$
$$800 \text{ calories} = 3500 \text{ kJ}$$
$$1500 \text{ calories} = 6000 \text{ kJ}$$
$$2500 \text{ calories} = 10\ 000 \text{ kJ}$$

1

DIET AND THE SUPPLY
OF ENERGY

THE FOOD WE EAT

The body is a machine that needs fuel, both to provide energy for activity and to maintain a temperature warmer than the atmosphere.
The body is never still and, even when we sleep, activity is continuous.
The heart is a pump that by its contractions drives blood through the
arteries seventy or eighty times every minute. The lungs are expand-
ing and contracting, and the bowel is writhing gently to propel the
food. In addition to these grosser movements the kidneys are excret-
ing urine and there is a constant flow of nutriments in and out of the
cells. Metabolism* is continuous and ceaseless. All this energy requires fuel and the food we eat is the fuel which is burned or metabolized in the oxygen we breathe.

There are three types of food, distinguished from each other by the
manner in which they are broken down and used by the tissues of the
body. Carbohydrate is the commonest food, the least expensive and
providing energy most readily. Protein is necessary for the nourishment and replacement of the cells and tissues of the body; it is in short
supply since its source is mainly animal and it is consequently more
expensive. Fat provides the body's reserve source of energy and in fact
represents the most compact type of fuel available. Unfortunately, it is
not easily assimilated and cannot be taken in large quantities without
nausea. Most diets today contain proportions of each of these three
types of food but the proportions vary considerably with such factors
as climate, availability, and racial habits. In cold countries the pro-

* Metabolism can be defined as the over-all sum of the chemical reactions occurring
in the body.

portion of fat is higher because of its heat-giving quality and because appetites are keener. In poor countries the diet is largely carbohydrate because this is cheaper and more readily available than protein.

Nobody is quite sure what food primitive man ate, though judging by the apes today it seems likely that he relied on the vegetable kingdom and was not primarily a carnivore. It was only when he learnt to use tools that he acquired his taste for animal flesh. The fact is, all three forms of food are potentially interchangeable. At the turn of the century numerous experiments were conducted on animals fed from birth with pure protein, pure carbohydrate, or even pure fat. Although the animals fed on pure carbohydrate, for example, did not necessarily flourish they were nevertheless able to build up normal muscle and tissues formed from protein. Even though the diet did not contain protein, the animal's metabolism enabled it to convert carbohydrate into protein and into fat.

TABLE 1.1   *Some minerals necessary in diet*

Mineral	Source	Metabolic role
Sodium	Common salt	Essential constituent body fluids
Calcium	Milk, cheese	Formation of bones and teeth
Fluorine	Water supply	Teeth enamel
Iron	Meat, eggs	Constituent of blood
Iodine	Water supply	Thyroid hormone

We are aware, of course, that the body cannot be kept in a state of health with protein, carbohydrate and fat alone. The diet must also contain adequate fluid and adequate mineral salts (see Table 1.1). Sodium and potassium must be available for the metabolism of the cells, adequate calcium is needed for the bones and teeth, iron is necessary for the production of blood, fluorine is needed to prevent dental decay, and iodine is needed for the proper functioning of the thyroid gland. But even with adequate fluid and adequate minerals, proper use will not be made of these components unless vitamins are present as well. Vitamins are factors present mostly in fresh food and have a specific action on various stages of the body's metabolism (see Table 1.2). Thus, without vitamin C the body is unable to use iron in the manufacture of haemoglobin, the constituent of the red cells which carries oxygen from the lungs.

TABLE 1.2 *Vitamins*

Type	Main source	Function
A	Animal fats, butter, cream, eggs, milk, cod-liver oil	Necessary for healthy vision
B	Cereals, nuts, yeast, eggs, liver, legumes	Essential for normal metabolism, functioning of nervous system and formation of blood
C	Fresh fruit and vegetables	Normal formation of blood and capillaries
D	Butter, eggs, milk, cod-liver oil	Regulates bone metabolism
K	Fish, liver, fruit, spinach	Regulates normal blood clotting mechanism

CARBOHYDRATE FOODS

The chief carbohydrate foods in Western countries are bread, cereals and potatoes. In Italy spaghetti heads the list, while in the vast continents of China and India rice is the staple diet. Most of these carbohydrate foods in modern times have been processed and refined so that we do not receive them in their natural state. White flour, for example, is made from wheat after the husk (bran) has been discarded. But the wheat bran is an important source of dietary fibre and fibre plays an essential role in digestion. Fibre is present in all parts of the structure of the growing plant and, when eaten, fibre is neither digested nor absorbed. Fibre absorbs and retains water in the bowel and this adds bulk to the bowel content. One of the commonest causes of constipation (and many other bowel disorders) is lack of fibre in the diet. Furthermore when fibre is present in food it delays the breakdown of carbohydrate and the absorption of glucose from the bowel.

Sugar is a type of carbohydrate, and the more civilized the country the higher the consumption of sugar per head. Sugar is in fact a highly concentrated and unnatural foodstuff and there is good evidence that our metabolism has never adequately adapted to the consumption of excessive sugar which is too rapidly absorbed and assimilated. Huge quantities of natural sugar-cane or beet are needed to produce only small amounts of sugar.*

Carbohydrates in general have to be broken down into smaller units before they can be absorbed by the bowel into the blood system. These smaller units are known as monosaccharides, and glucose is the most basic and most important monosaccharide. Ordinary sugar consists of two monosaccharides so that when sugar is taken the normal processes of digestion and assimilation are largely circumvented. When we ingest bread or potato, digestion starts in the mouth. The starch is split by the enzymes from the salivary glands so that as the food is chewed, digestion is already beginning. When the bolus of food is swallowed into the stomach, the acid of the stomach further reduces some types of carbohydrate to monosaccharides, but the primary site of carbohydrate digestion lies in the small intestine when the partly digested food has left the stomach. Here enzymatic juices pour into the bowel by a duct leading from the pancreas gland. All the remaining carbohydrates are hydrolysed by these enzymes to monosaccharides and particularly to glucose. Carbohydrates now converted to glucose can be absorbed by the cells of the intestinal wall and so into the bloodstream. Glucose is the body's readiest form of energy. When glucose is transported to the liver, it is broken down and metabolized with the production of heat and energy. The liver is the largest organ in the body and lies under the right diaphragm in the upper abdomen. It is the metabolic mill which consumes the various units of food brought to it by the bloodstream.

After a meal, and particularly one containing sugar, there is a rapid absorption of glucose into the blood. The blood always contains some circulating sugar and this blood sugar always temporarily increases after a meal. However, there is an extraordinarily efficient mechanism by which the amount of sugar in the blood varies very little. As the sugar in the blood starts to increase after a meal, because of increased absorption from the bowel, the liver is capable of absorbing it and storing excess in an inert form known as glycogen. The remainder is metabolized to provide energy. The degree to which the liver can store

* The biochemical term for ordinary sugar is sucrose. Sucrose is a combination of glucose and fructose, and it is glucose which is present in the bloodstream. We use the term 'sugar' to include glucose and strictly speaking blood sugar means blood glucose. Dextrose is a form of glucose and is absorbed and metabolized in the same way as glucose.

glycogen is not limitless. Constant overeating, particularly of sweet foods containing sugar, leads to satiation of the liver's store of glycogen. Alternative methods of storage must now be used. By various metabolic pathways in the liver, excess glucose is ultimately transformed to fat and deposited as fat stores in the subcutaneous tissues. Plainly, overeating of sugar inevitably leads to obesity.

TABLE 1.3 *Some important hormones*

Hormone	Gland	Main action
Insulin	Pancreas	Lowers blood sugar
*Glucagon	Pancreas	Raises blood sugar
*Growth hormone	Pituitary	Enhances growth
*Thyroxin	Thyroid	Stimulates metabolism
Parathormone	Parathyroids	Controls calcium metabolism
*Cortisol	Adrenals	Controls inflammatory reactions
*Adrenalin	Adrenals	Prepares response to stress
Androgens	Testicles	Male hormone
Oestrogens	Ovaries	Female hormone

* All these hormones tend to cause a rise in blood sugar and so counteract the effect of insulin.

The mechanism by which sugar in the blood is kept at a constant level is a most complex and intricate one and is mediated through a series of hormones (see Table 1.3). Hormones are chemical activators which control various metabolic activities and are produced by a series of glands or organs. These are placed in different sites in the body. For example, the thyroid gland, which produces thyroxin, lies in the neck. The adrenal glands, which produce cortisol, lie perched above the kidneys. There are at least four different hormones which by their actions increase the amount of sugar in the blood, but there is only one hormone which will bring down the level of sugar in the blood. This hormone is insulin and it is produced by the pancreas gland. Surprisingly, the cells which produce insulin are scattered throughout the pancreas gland in little isolated clumps known as islets. The rest of the gland contains cells which produce enzymes necessary for the digestion of food in the bowel and which are poured into the bowel through the pancreatic duct. Insulin enters the bloodstream directly from the islet cells and its sole purpose seems to be that of encouraging glucose to enter into the liver. Without insulin, sugar accumulates in the blood and normal metabolism is delayed or distorted as will be described later.

PROTEIN

Protein foods are primarily needed for the replacement of normal body wear and tear and for the growth of new tissues. The main sources of protein are the muscles of animals, birds and fish, and also milk, cheese and eggs. Protein is also accessible from non-animal sources, particularly peas and beans. The soya bean is a helpful source of protein in countries where meat is not freely available. Although the body is capable of producing protein from carbohydrate and fat, its ability to do so is limited and unless the diet contains a minimum of protein serious disease must ensue.

The digestion of protein begins in the stomach when the gastric enzyme, pepsin, breaks down the large protein molecule to smaller units known as peptides. When food passes from the stomach to the intestine, further breakdown of peptides occurs under the influence of enzymes from the pancreas. The smallest units, known as the amino-acids, are now in a form suitable for absorption by the intestine into the blood stream whence they are transported to the liver. Amino-acids are now incorporated into the metabolic mill, where they can be built up again to peptides and proteins, appropriate to the body's needs.

FATS

Fats form an important energy food and a highly concentrated form of body fuel. The principal source of fat in the normal diet is from butter and margarine, or as oils and lard used in cooking. Cream and meat fat are also common sources of this food. The amount of fat in the diet varies a great deal. In cold countries more fat is eaten than in the tropics, while men involved in heavy work usually need a higher fat intake.

Fat is mostly digested in the small intestine. No material change in fat structure takes place in the mouth or in the stomach, but when fat leaves the stomach the globules are emulsified by bile transmitted to

the bowel from the gall bladder. After this first stage, further breakdown of fat is mediated by the pancreatic juices whose enzymes con-

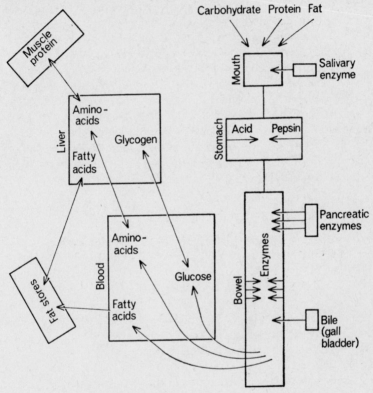

FIG. 1.1. Diagrammatic representation of food metabolism

vert fat into smaller units known as glycerides and fatty acids. These
can now be absorbed by the small intestine into the lymphatic system
and thence into the bloodstream. Fatty acids and glycerides are deposited in the fat depots, mostly under the skin, and are stored as neutral
fats. In the past, fat was regarded as an inert store only used for body
metabolism in times of stress. However, recent studies have shown
this attitude to be erroneous. In fact, body fat is in a ceaseless state of
flux. It is constantly being broken down to fatty acids and carried to
the liver. At the same time new fatty acids from the liver are constantly

being incorporated into the fatty stores. Indeed, there is accumulating evidence that fat plays a most important role in the body's metabolism and may rival carbohydrate as the prime source of energy. This is not altogether surprising when we realise how concentrated fat is as a source of energy. A gramme of fat produces more energy than a gramme of carbohydrate and a gramme of protein put together.

Cholesterol is a product of fat metabolism and is carried in the blood in the form of lipoprotein. Fats derived from animal sources (butter, lard, cream) lead to an increase in blood cholesterol, whereas fats from vegetable sources (corn oil, sunflower oil) are much less prone to do so. Excess cholesterol present in the blood can be deposited in the lining of the arteries and can dispose to thickening and narrowing of these arteries. This is the reason for advising restriction of animal fats in the diet.

FORMATION OF A DIET

In building up a suitable diet for the growth of a child or the maintenance of health in an adult, various principles must be borne in mind. The diet must be adequate in quantity. It must provide enough energy and it must keep the body weight at a suitable level. In starvation muscle is lost, fat stores are depleted, and the sugar in the blood ultimately falls to too low a level. If excess food is eaten, the fat stores become over-replete and there is a tendency for too much sugar to accumulate in the blood, with resultant diabetes.

The amount of food necessary to maintain health cannot be assessed by its mere weight. In the assessment of the value of food the unit to be considered is that of calories. A calorie is the measure of the amount of heat given off when a unit of food is oxidized, just as the value of coal can be measured by its yield of heat when it is burned. Some foods have an extremely low yield of calories and these are mostly described as roughage. Thus, cabbage provides bulk in the diet but with the production of very few calories. In fact, a diet that is too concentrated and contains too little roughage provides poor stimulus to bowel movement and may lead to constipation. If ever the day dawns when we can provide all the calories needed in the form of pills, artificial roughage will have to be added.

The three main components of food, carbohydrate, protein and fat, all produce their own standard rate of calories when metabolized. A gramme of carbohydrate and a gramme of protein each yields 4 cal, while a gramme of fat produces 9 cal. In order to maintain good health a minimum of 1200 cal is needed daily, though this would be quite inadequate for most adults leading an active life. A healthy male performing a heavy job may use from 3000 to 5000 cal without laying down excessive fat, whereas a sedentary worker may only require 2000 cal. The calorie intake varies enormously from person to person, and the factors which determine individual requirements are not really understood. Of course, broadly speaking it is clear enough that some people eat too much and become fat as a result. In others appetite is poor, not enough food is taken and weight is lost. However, considerations of this sort beg the question of the meaning of appetite.

Much study and experimentation have been undertaken to find what it is that determines appetite. Some people never seem to be satisfied however much food they eat, while others appear quite indifferent to food. Evidence has accumulated that there is a centre in the brain (in the hypothalamus) which controls the desire to eat food. In experimental animals in which the appetite centre in the hypothalamus has been damaged, the animals eat so voraciously and insistently that ultimately they increase their weight threefold with enormous deposition of fat. There is no evidence of damage to this hypothalamic centre in men who become obese and nothing to suggest that enormously fat people have any disorder of the hypothalamus. Consequently, although we suspect that excessive greed may be due to a disorder of the hypothalamic centre, as suggested by this experimental evidence, no direct proof of this sort has been produced in man.

Naturally, many social factors affect the appetite. If we live in an affluent society with food freely available and made tempting by expert cooking, obesity is much more likely to be prevalent than when food is scarce. Furthermore, in modern life food can be concentrated in a highly unnatural way in the form of sugar. Sugar yields an enormously high calorie content with subsequent deposition of fat. In addition to these factors, clearly there must be individual variations in dealing with food. It is commonplace experience that some people seem to eat voraciously and remain quite thin, while others put on weight even with a modest intake of food. In this respect, it is worth remembering that once a person has overeaten and become obese it requires only a normal intake of food to maintain the weight at that level. Let us say that during pregnancy a woman, spending a good deal of time at home surrounded by food, easily bored, has taken to considerable overeating. She may put on several stones in weight. Although thereafter her dietary intake is modest, she will remain obese. Only by a programme of near starvation will she be able to get rid of the excess put on during her pregnancy.

In determining the ideal number of calories for an individual, the aim is to achieve the ideal weight for the subject's age, height and frame, and this ideal weight can be obtained from charts prepared for this purpose. There is no heaven-sent description of an ideal weight. All we can do is to look at the expectation of life at different weight levels and decide which weight carries with it the best expectation of longevity. This is an actuarial exercise. Having decided the number of calories required under the circumstances prevailing, we can then work out the proportions of carbohydrate, protein and fat required to produce the desired number of calories. In an adult, an intake of 75 g of protein daily is necessary for good health, and since each gramme of protein provides 4 cal this means 300 cal a day from protein. A reasonable carbohydrate intake would be 300 g a day, providing 1200 cal. The amount of fat is restricted by its palatability and 100 g is usually all that need be taken, providing a further 900 cal. Thus, a diet of 75 g protein, 300 g carbohydrate and 100 g fat will yield a diet providing 2400 cal. If chocolates, jams and sugar are added to the diet, immediately the total calorie intake goes shooting up and quickly exceeds all metabolic requirements.

In deciding how to provide the various amounts of protein, carbohydrate and fat, we must resort to appropriate tables which give the constitution of common articles of food. The percentage of protein, carbohydrate and fat in such common articles of food as milk, cheese and meat must be known as must the weights in ounces or in grammes of each type of food taken in each day. With these facts to hand it is easy to draw up a list of common foods available for each meal and, knowing the proportions of protein, carbohydrate and fat that each contain, it is possible to work out the amount of calories we eat during an ordinary day. A well-balanced diet will not only have an adequate quantity of calories but also adequate fresh food to provide vitamins, foods to provide minerals, and adequate roughage to promote bowel function. In providing a diet for a particular individual, it is good practice to find out what is normally eaten and to use this as a basis. It is no good working out a diet in terms of bread and potatoes for someone who has never eaten anything but rice.

Mention has been made of the importance of roughage in the diet and indeed the quality of carbohydrate is every bit as important as the quantity. Dietary fibre derives from plant structures and is present in all parts of the plant. Thus fruit, vegetables and salads all contain fibre and so does natural wheat and rice. Unfortunately modern methods of refining flour and rice discard the outer husk (bran) and so deprives white bread and polished rice of almost all its fibre content. This refinement leads to at least two harmful effects. Firstly, the purified carbohydrate is broken down and converted to glucose too rapidly in the bowel: and secondly, the lack of bulk in the content of the bowel leads to constipation and other intestinal disorders. To avoid these troubles, wholemeal bread and brown rice should be used. Cakes and biscuits should be made from wholemeal flour and should not be sweetened with sugar: natural fruit can be used for flavouring. Many cereals are available (particularly All-Bran) which have a high fibre content, and indeed bran itself can be added to the diet if constipation is troublesome. Plenty of fruit, vegetables and salads should also be taken. Since this type of food is bulky and satisfies the appetite, it is unlikely that the total calorie content will be excessive from these sources.

DISORDERS OF METABOLISM

As will be explained, in the disorder known as diabetes there is a relative lack of the hormone insulin. The immediate effect of this lack is that glucose absorbed from the bowel is no longer available as a source of energy to the liver or to the muscles. Without insulin, the liver is unable to assimilate glucose and so proceeds to break down its stores of glycogen with the production of even more glucose. Excessive amounts of glucose appear in the blood, inaccessible for the purpose of the body's metabolism. Other sources of energy must now be sought and the liver must utilize fatty acids as an alternative. Fat is broken down to fatty acids and the flow of fatty acids to the liver is vastly increased to meet this new demand. The normal conversion of glucose to fat is inhibited and imperfect products of excessive fat metabolism begin to appear. These products are known as ketones, and their appearance immediately suggests an inadequate metabolism of carbohydrate and of fat. Ketones are toxic compounds and their accumulation in the blood leads to excessive acidification.

Protein is equally involved in this deranged metabolism. The liver attempts to derive glucose from the breakdown of amino-acids and this, in turn, means that the body is deprived of its protein stores. There is a failure to rebuild tissue protein from its natural sources.

The sum total of a lack of insulin and the failure to utilize glucose properly is the accumulation of sugar and ketones in the blood, with the deprivation of fats and of proteins. In a subject deprived of insulin by destruction of the pancreas, there is a loss of weight due to diminution of the fat stores and wasting of muscle, a loss of strength due to inadequate utilization of glucose and a whole series of secondary effects following the accumulation of ketones and glucose in the blood.

Normally after a meal is eaten, the sugar in the blood does not exceed 120 mg for every 100 ml of blood. Above this level insulin gets to work and more glucose is taken up by the liver and muscles. An hour or so after a meal, the sugar in the blood has fallen to about 80 mg and this is the sort of level maintained overnight. When the sugar in the blood vastly exceeds this level, as happens in diabetes, the concentration of glucose affects the secretion of urine by the kidney and sugar appears in the urine. It is as if sugar spills over into the urine from the blood when it exceeds a certain concentration and indeed we refer to the level at which this occurs as the 'renal threshold'. Normally the renal threshold is about 180 mg/100 ml, and the appearance of sugar in the urine means that the blood level has exceeded this figure. In diabetes, the level of sugar in the blood may far exceed 180 mg and consequently sugar is found in the urine. The kidney can only get rid of this excess sugar when it is in solution, so that large quantities of urine must be passed to get rid of the unusable sugar. In short, the patient is constantly passing urine to get rid of excess sugar in the blood and, since the fluid must be replaced, he is constantly thirsty. The presence of ketones in the blood suggesting improper fat metabolism also leads to secondary effects.

Acidification of the blood by ketones causes excessive over-

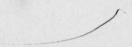

breathing. The breath contains carbonic acid and this mechanism helps to restore the normal blood acidity. In addition, ketones can be excreted in the breath and in the urine. Characteristically, in severe diabetes the breathing is laboured, the breath smells of ketones (acetone) and the urine gives a positive reaction when tested for ketones. The smell of acetone in the breath is sweet and sickly and has often been likened to new-mown hay. This represents a serious deterioration of body metabolism. In clinical terms, the patient is wasted due to lack of fat and protein, he is excessively tired, he is constantly thirsty, his breath smells of ketones (acetone) and his extremities are cold. If this disorder is not corrected, excessive accumulation of sugar and ketones in the blood leads to coma and in the days before insulin was available this condition was universally fatal. Happily today this state of affairs is seldom seen. Administration of insulin obtained from the pancreas glands of animals soon leads to restoration of normal metabolism.

2

DIAGNOSIS AND ORIGIN
OF DIABETES

WHAT IS DIABETES?

The diagnosis of diabetes depends on the level of sugar in the blood. This definition immediately poses difficulties because there is considerable variation in blood sugar levels in normal people. For example, the blood sugar rises normally after a meal and falls again when we are fasting. Usually, in the fasting state on rising in the morning, the amount of sugar in the blood is about 80 mg/100 ml, but after breakfast this may rise to 120 mg/100 ml. Normally, the blood sugar seldom exceeds 160 mg/100 ml even after eating a heavy meal containing a lot of sugar. In diabetes, the blood sugar is elevated above normal and usually exceeds 200 mg/100 ml. However, there is no precise point at which it is possible to say that diabetes is present since occasionally blood sugars may temporarily rise above normal levels. Some help in the diagnosis may be given by testing the urine.

URINE TESTS

Sugar does not appear in the urine under ordinary circumstances until the level of sugar in the blood exceeds 180 mg/100 ml. When the sugar in the blood exceeds this level, sugar starts to appear in the urine. Consequently one of the first tests to reveal diabetes is the examination of the urine for sugar. If the urine shows sugar, then it is suggestive that the blood sugar is elevated and diabetes is the cause. This test is by no means completely reliable. The level at which sugar appears in the urine does not always accurately reflect the level of sugar in the blood. Sugar is excreted from the blood into the urine by the kidney and the level of blood sugar at which the kidney excretes sugar into the blood is called the renal threshold. The renal threshold is usually 180 mg of sugar in each 100 ml blood, but in some people the threshold may be very much lower, perhaps only 100 mg/100 ml. In such people with a low renal threshold, sugar appears in the urine even though the blood sugars are normal. This is an entirely innocent condition though it proves to be a nuisance at insurance examinations since the presence of sugar in the urine suggests the possibility of diabetes. On the other hand, the renal threshold may be abnormally high. In this case, although the sugar in the blood is raised to diabetic levels, no sugar appears in the urine. Since a high blood sugar is deleterious to health, absence of sugar in the urine may mean a delay in the discovery of diabetes and a delay in necessary treatment. Hence, the testing for sugar in the urine is only helpful if the renal threshold is known. Routine testing of the urine in the general population has shown that the presence or absence of sugar in the urine is an unreliable method of diagnosing the presence of diabetes. Its presence increases the possibilities of diabetes but its absence does not exclude it absolutely.

Thanks to modern techniques, the testing of sugar in the urine is now extremely simple. Two methods are freely available. The first is by using Clinitest tablets. Ten drops of water are added to five drops of urine in a test tube and a tablet is added. The tablet generates its own heat and the solution boils. If no sugar is present in the urine, the colour is a clear blue, but if sugar is present, the solution changes to green or orange according to the amount of sugar present. This method of testing the urine gives a rough quantitative guide to the amount of sugar present. This method is most valuable in diabetics taking insulin when it is important to know how much sugar is present. The second method is the Clinistix test in which an impregnated strip is dipped into the urine. If no sugar is present, the strip colour remains pink whereas if sugar is in the urine the colour turns to purple. This is a more sensitive test as to whether or not sugar is present in the urine, but it is no guide as to the quantity. Consequently, Clinistix is most useful in deciding whether or not the urine contains sugar but is not helpful in showing how much sugar is present.

The diagnosis of diabetes may be suspected by the presence of symptoms, but very often the patient may not feel unwell and suspicion may have been roused by the finding of sugar in the urine on a routine insurance examination. Consequently, some method must be used to define exactly whether or not diabetes is present. The commonest test in this respect is called the glucose tolerance test, and depends on the fate of glucose after it has been taken by mouth in a measured quantity. The sugar in the blood is measured at intervals after the subject has drunk a test solution containing 50 g glucose in the morning without having had any previous food or drink. The blood sugars are estimated in the fasting state and subsequently half an hour, one hour, one and a half hours, and finally two hours after the glucose has been taken. Normally the amount of sugar in the blood in the fasting state should not exceed 90 mg/100 ml. It should not rise above 160 mg/100 ml after glucose has been absorbed, and it should fall again to less than 100 mg/100 ml two hours later. In other words, in normal people the glucose load is rapidly assimilated by the action of insulin, and after two hours it has all been stored in the liver and muscles as glycogen. In diabetes, the fasting level exceeds 80 mg and after the glucose has been taken the sugar in the blood continues to increase, often failing to fall at all even after two hours. In short, the body is entirely unable to store away the sugar when it has been absorbed.

In theory then the glucose tolerance curve offers a precise diagnosis of diabetes. In practice, anomalies arise. Whereas in overt cases the type of glucose tolerance curve is constantly abnormal, in borderline cases where only one or two of the blood sugars are raised, variations in the curve may occur under different circumstances. For example, the ability to assimilate glucose becomes impaired after a period of starvation and a temporarily abnormal curve may be obtained in normal people who have deliberately undereaten for the days preceding the test. Nor are the curves necessarily reproducible. A slightly abnormal curve one day may be quite normal when it is repeated a few weeks later. The most important difficulty lies with these borderline cases. Gross abnormalities are always indicative of diabetes and a completely normal curve always excludes the diagnosis. The curve in which one or two points are abnormal offer diagnostic difficulties since we are not quite sure whether or not these patients ultimately deteriorate and progress to overt diabetes, or whether they return to normal. Usually, if the curve is a borderline one, it is wise to repeat it after a few months.

Another important finding is that the ability to assimilate a glucose load deteriorates with age and when glucose tolerance tests are performed in men and women over the age of 70, the majority of them show abnormalities in the blood sugar curve consistent with a diagnosis of diabetes. If this is the sole criterion in the diagnosis, we would reach the astonishing conclusion that the majority of elderly people have diabetes. Clearly our present methods of defining diabetes leave something to be desired, but the real issue is not so much in the delineation of the diagnosis of diabetes but whether these minor abnormalities are of any ultimate significance as far as the health of the individual is concerned. This is a matter of considerable interest and speculation. Evidence is accruing that the higher the blood sugar, the greater the tendency to hardening of the arteries and coronary thrombosis.

INSULIN IN THE BLOOD

Following the discovery in 1921 that the raised sugar in the blood in diabetes could be corrected by injections of insulin, it was naturally assumed that diabetes was due to lack of insulin. However, no methods were available at that time for measuring the amount of insulin produced by the pancreas in normal people or in diabetics. In the 1950s, methods became available for measuring the level of insulin circulating in the blood and in recent years these techniques have become more accurate and reliable. Many surprises were in store. It soon became apparent that whereas young thin diabetics produced very little insulin, mildly obese diabetics produced large quantities of insulin, indeed more than normal people. These puzzling facts needed explanation.

Experimental evidence obtained in animals suggested that although insulin was normally produced, it could be rendered inactive by various antagonists present in the blood. Such antagonists to insulin were found in the blood of diabetics and were not present in the blood of non-diabetic subjects. For a time these findings led to the theory that diabetes developed not because the pancreas failed to produce insulin, but because some factor in the blood prevented insulin from performing its normal duties. Controversy still exists as to the nature and practical importance of these antagonists, but continuing experience in measuring insulin production in normal subjects has made at least one dilemma easier to understand. This is the discovery that the highest production of insulin occurs in obesity, irrespective of whether diabetes is present or not. Estimations of insulin in the blood in really fat people reveal levels many times higher than in normal non-obese subjects. The explanation for this finding is under investigation but it seems likely that a high level of insulin is necessary to deal with excessive eating and subsequent storage of fat. Obese diabetics also have a high level of insulin but not so high as obese subjects without diabetes. In other words, it may be that diabetes occurs in obesity because the pancreas is no longer able to maintain a continuously high output of insulin. Although large quantities of insulin are indeed produced, the amount is inadequate for the dual task of laying down fat, and of storing excess sugar as glycogen. Hence, sugar accumulates in the blood despite the presence of high levels of insulin and diabetes ensues.

In children or in thin diabetics, insulin may be found in the blood when the condition is first diagnosed. There is not as much as in fat diabetics but still as much or even more than in normal, lean, non-diabetics. At the time of diagnosis these patients have very high levels of sugar in the blood. A raised level of sugar in the blood is the most potent stimulus to the production of insulin from the pancreas. In a normal healthy adult, injections of glucose into the blood stimulates a tremendous release of insulin from the pancreas. If the level of sugar in the blood is artificially raised by the continuous infusion of a glucose solution into a vein, the output of insulin increases enormously. The raised level of insulin in newly diagnosed young diabetics must be seen in this context. Whereas the level of insulin is above normal, it is far less than the level the normal subject would produce if faced with a similarly high blood sugar level. In short, although the child who develops diabetes may show an elevated level of insulin in the blood, it is entirely inappropriate to the stimulus of the high blood sugar level. The current concept is that in these cases there is a relative and gradual failure of insulin production and this leads to an increasing inadequacy of glucose storage. The sugar in the blood gradually rises and stimulates the pancreas to produce more insulin. As the gland is unable fully to respond to this stimulus, the blood sugar rises further. Ultimately then, we reach a stage where the blood sugar is constantly elevated though insulin is still present. Hence, we believe that in young, thin diabetics the basic defect lies in the inability of the islet cells of the pancreas to produce adequate quantities of insulin.

BIG BABIES

One of the most puzzling aspects of diabetes is that women prone to develop this complaint often produce large babies many years before the actual development of diabetes. It is not uncommon for a woman to develop diabetes at the age of 60 and to reveal that her two sons born some 40 years previously both weighed more than 10 lb at birth.

There is also a higher incidence of stillborn babies in mothers who later develop diabetes. Here again, the stillborn baby is often large and grossly overweight. These findings strongly suggest that some abnormality exists in these women long before diabetes itself is manifest. The most stringent metabolic tests on women who have large babies fail to demonstrate any certain abnormality of glucose tolerance or carbohydrate metabolic disorder. Nevertheless, some disorder must exist in a high proportion of these women since they ultimately develop diabetes. This problem is a very basic one for it suggests that there is much more to diabetes than a raised level of blood sugar. When the pancreas glands of these stillborn babies are examined, usually the insulin-producing islet cells are grossly enlarged, as if they were trying to compensate for some maternal inadequacy. This intriguing problem has been the source of much research but so far no satisfying solution has been reached.

TYPES OF DIABETES

Although in the large majority of cases the cause of diabetes remains obscure, there are patients in whom the onset of diabetes is secondary to some other disorder. These cases are known as secondary diabetes. For example, a tumour or growth of the pancreas gland may necessitate pancreatectomy, or removal of the pancreas by surgical operation. In such cases, since there is no production of insulin, diabetes inevitably results. The pancreas can also be destroyed by various disorders which lead to fibrosis, or scarring of all the islet cells of the pancreas, as may occur in an ailment known as haemochromatosis. Here too, diabetes inevitably results as a secondary effect of islet cell destruction.

Several hormones antagonize the action of insulin and if these are produced in excess, the effect of insulin may be swamped and diabetes will result. As will be seen in Table 1.3, at least five hormones counteract the effect of insulin and so lead to abnormal elevation of the level of sugar in the blood. Excessive production of growth hormone leads to a condition called gigantism, when this occurs before puberty, and acromegaly when it happens in the adult. Growth hormone is produced by the pituitary gland, a small bean-shaped organ lying below the brain. It is responsible for the growth and development of the child and, if it fails, the child fails to grow and remains a perpetual Peter Pan. If the reverse occurs and excessive growth hormone is produced by the pituitary, the child grows to an excessive height, perhaps over 7 ft tall. Since growth hormone antagonizes the effect of insulin, a high proportion of these giants develop diabetes. If excess growth hormone occurs in the adult, the condition of acromegaly appears in which the features become coarse and thickened and the hands and feet become steadily broader and larger. Here again, about a third of patients with acromegaly develop diabetes due to elevation of the blood sugar by excess growth hormone.

Another hormone which antagonizes insulin is cortisol. Cortisol is produced by the adrenal glands. These organs lie above the kidneys and, if they overact, excess cortisol leads to high blood pressure and diabetes. Cortisol damps down the effects of inflammation and is prescribed in tablet form to patients suffering from various inflammatory ailments, such as rheumatism or asthma. In such patients, if the dose of cortisol is too high or if treatment is prolonged, diabetes is liable to occur, since the action of insulin is suppressed.

Of much interest in recent years has been the demonstration that the contraceptive pill leads to a deterioration of glucose tolerance. If the glucose tolerance test is performed in women starting the pill and is then repeated after about a year, the blood sugar levels after taking glucose are somewhat higher than those taken originally. In other words, the pill creates a tendency towards diabetes. In practice, it is quite unusual for those taking the pill ever to develop actual diabetes and it can be argued that the changes in glucose tolerance are of no material significance in the vast majority of women taking these preparations for contraceptive purposes. The pill contains an oestrogenic compound, a synthetic preparation of the natural hormone produced by the ovaries, and it is probably this hormone which exerts this effect. It is well known that oestrogens tend to lead to an increase in weight and this in itself might impair glucose tolerance, but the effect is not confined to those women who put on weight. At most it could be said that in women with a tendency to diabetes, taking the pill could make matters worse.

Apart from hormones, some drugs given for the treatment of various ailments may damage the islet cells and inhibit production of insulin. This is particularly true of the chlorothiazide group of diuretics. Diuretics are given to increase the output of fluid from the body and are of special value in heart disease when the circulation is impaired. The body may become waterlogged due to this circulatory failure and swelling of the legs occurs. Diuretics encourage an increased output of fluid by the kidneys and so are enormously helpful in relieving congestion due to the impairment of the circulation. However, an unfortunate effect is that diabetes may result, since chlorothiazide causes gradual suppression of the islet cell production of insulin. This is a small price to pay for the improvement that diuretics can give to patients with heart trouble.

In the vast majority of diabetics, no cause can be found for the onset of their ailment. In young people, it is often suspected that there may have been mechanical destruction of the islet cells by a virus infection and, rarely, diabetes has been known to follow an attack of mumps. Mostly, however, no such evidence exists.

For the purposes of classification, diabetes can be divided into two types:

1. *Mild diabetes* occurring in middle-aged people, frequently associated with obesity. In this type of diabetes, symptoms are usually mild or nonexistent so that the diagnosis is often made by the chance finding of sugar in the urine at a routine medical examination. Once the diagnosis is confirmed, these patients are easily restored to normal health by a reduction of food intake. This relieves the demands placed on the pancreas. Production of insulin becomes adequate to store

excess sugar as glycogen, since it no longer has to lay down excess deposition of fat. If simple restriction of diet is not enough, tablets may be given which stimulate the pancreas to produce more insulin. Usually, diabetes of this sort is easy to control and with a co-operative patient the expectation of life and health should not be unduly impaired.

The urine contains sugar but only rarely contains acetone. Consequently, diabetic coma is very unusual in this type of patient.

2. *Severe diabetes* can occur at any age but is typified by that occurring in children or young people. The onset of diabetes in these cases is generally more sudden and the symptoms, which are dealt with later, much more severe. These patients have lost a lot of weight and are usually very thin. The urine contains sugar and, what is more significant, acetone as well. Without insulin, expectation of life would be very restricted and coma would soon ensue. These are the patients to whom insulin offers health and activity.

Although these two types of diabetes may seem quite different, no clear delineation can in fact be made. A mild obese diabetic woman can have a child who develops acute diabetes. They are differentiated by their need for insulin. Thin, young diabetics invariably need insulin, whereas it is quite exceptional for obese diabetics to need it.

HEREDITY IN DIABETES

It is generally accepted that diabetes is an hereditary ailment and tends to run in families. However, the degree to which the ailment is inherited has been open to a great deal of discussion in recent years. To begin with, it does not seem to be that diabetes is necessarily a single disorder easy to define. The borderline between normality and diabetes is ill-defined. As has already been pointed out, the older we get the less perfect is the mechanism for storing away sugar. In elderly people, diabetes is very much more common than in the younger generation so that age itself is an important contributing factor. Also, as we have seen, diabetes may be caused by destruction of the pancreas mechanically, by drugs, or by overaction of other hormones. In such cases, there is clearly an inter-play of various factors and perhaps the most important of these factors is simple obesity. Obesity places a great stress on the islet cell production of insulin and diabetes is very much more common in those who are overweight. Consequently, it is not always easy to disentangle hereditary factors from those caused by other ailments or by environmental stresses. In fact, it is by no means clear what is inherited. Diabetes may result from an impoverished production of insulin by the pancreas but this in itself may be the result of many different factors within the islets leading to this reduction of insulin. It seems reasonable to conclude that some deficiency in the mechanism of insulin production may be inherited but that diabetes only results when a combination of effects leads to an actual breakdown.

The evidence that diabetes runs in families can be found by questioning those patients who develop diabetes as to whether or not any of their family suffer from this complaint. When this is done it seems that more than a third of those developing diabetes have someone in their family who also has diabetes. This is a much higher percentage than is obtained when subjects without diabetes are similarly questioned. In such people about only one in twenty know of a diabetic relative.

Interesting studies have been carried out on identical twins. These are twins formed by the splitting of a single fertilized ovum at the time of conception and differs from dissimilar twins where two separate ova are fertilized simultaneously. Identical twins are hard to distinguish by appearance, are always of the same sex and often have a similar mental attitude. There have now been many such twins where one of the pair develops diabetes. After a variable length of time, in about half of such cases, the other twin also develops the same ailment. This seems strong evidence of an inherited defect which is responsible for the development of diabetes though environmental factors may influence the actual time of onset. Apart from identical twins, there are many families where diabetes is particularly common and where several brothers and sisters all develop the complaint at an early age. Here, the hereditary factors must be particularly strong or multiple.

Despite all these findings, some two-thirds of those who develop diabetes have no family history of this complaint, so that heredity may not usually be very potent. If it were so, we would certainly expect diabetes to occur in nearly all the children born to couples both of whom are diabetics. In fact, the incidence of diabetes in the offspring of parents both of whom have diabetes is surprisingly low. Only about 5 per cent of the children born to such couples develop diabetes, and although this is a much higher incidence than in the population at large, it does not lend support to the idea that the inherited defect is a very dominating one. Put the other way round, if a diabetic girl marries a diabetic boy, the chances of their children having diabetes is only about one in twenty. A further comfort is that the offspring destined to develop diabetes may not do so until late in life and the diabetes may be very mild. If only one parent has diabetes, the chances of the children having diabetes is very small indeed and no diabetic need be deterred from having children on these grounds. Although as has been said, there are occasional families with the very frequent development of diabetes such families are quite exceptional.

Thus, although heredity plays a part in the development of diabetes, usually many other factors are equally important and no diabetic need fear to have children on the grounds that they too may develop diabetes. In those who have a family history of diabetes, the most important rule to deter development of the complaint is to be modest in eating and to avoid obesity.

3

SYMPTOMS OF DIABETES

⟨⟨⟨⟨⟩⟩⟩⟩

SYMPTOMS OF DIABETES

The exact moment of onset of diabetes can never be clearly defined and indeed there is no clear dividing line between normality and diabetes. As has been mentioned, the ability to store away excess sugar is gradually lost with increasing age so that if a definition of diabetes acceptable in younger people is applied to the older generation, we reach the absurd conclusion that the majority of people over 70 have diabetes. Since the inability to store away excess glucose may be a gradual process, symptoms may be equally insidious. Indeed, in middle age diabetes is frequently diagnosed as a result of a routine examination of the urine which reveals the presence of sugar. In many such cases, even when the diagnosis of diabetes is confirmed by glucose tolerance tests, the patient will not admit to any abnormal symptoms even on direct questioning. In children the situation is quite different. Here diabetes seems to come on much more quickly and symptoms may occur with increasing intensity. Since children seldom complain about their health, it often happens that a child is on the way to coma before the parents observe anything amiss.

The cardinal symptoms of diabetes are those of thirst, polyuria, loss of weight, and loss of energy.

THIRST

Thirst is a symptom often difficult to evaluate. We all of us experience thirst after unusual exercise or in hot weather due to excessive loss of moisture in the sweat and breath. Eating salty foods induces thirst.

Consequently it is common to ignore thirst as a symptom, since there is a tendency to ascribe it to something unusual in the food or in the weather. In well-developed diabetes, however, thirst can reach very severe proportions with the patient drinking as much as 10 or 12 pints a day. More significantly, in a severe case thirst may interrupt sleep and patients may start to leave a jug of water by the bedside at night. One such patient who worked as a bus conductress used to take a suitcase with four vacuum flasks of lemonade for each route. The situation can be exacerbated if the fluid which is drunk contains glucose, since this further increases the sugar in the blood. The thirst may be associated with a sticky unpleasant taste in the mouth. Sometimes thirst is associated with a feeling of hunger and characteristically this hunger is not appeased when food is taken.

POLYURIA

Polyuria, or the passing of large quantities of urine, is due to the body's effort to get rid of excess sugar from the blood and is the direct cause of the large intake of fluid. In children it often leads the parent to take the child to the doctor. Passing water frequently is not quite the same as polyuria. Frequency of micturition may be due to an infection of the bladder (cystitis) and irritation of the bladder leads to the need for frequent emptying. In this case, although the bladder is emptied frequently, the amount of urine passed is small. In diabetes, the bladder is not only emptied frequently but also large quantities of urine are passed each time. It may be noticed that the urine is very pale in colour since it is very diluted. Sometimes in men flecks of urine lead to small deposits of sugar on the shoes, appearing as white spots. One patient actually returned his shoes to the shop on the grounds that the leather was faulty. Sleep may be disturbed by the need to empty the bladder and here again this symptom must be differentiated from that occurring in older men in whom the prostate gland is enlarged. This causes bladder irritation, but the amount of urine passed may be small and the stream of urine restricted.

LOSS OF WEIGHT

One of the paradoxes of diabetes is that whereas obesity is one of the predisposing causes of diabetes, when the diabetes actually occurs the patient is pleased to find that the weight is no longer increasing. However, the loss of weight in this instance is not a healthy sign for it represents not only loss of fat but also loss of muscle in the form of sugar. In children or young people, loss of weight is gradual and insidious in the early stages so that parents may not be aware of what is happening. A relative who has not seen the child for some time is more likely to be struck by the thin, emaciated appearance.

LOSS OF ENERGY

Tiredness is a most difficult symptom to delineate since everybody feels tired from time to time and some people feel tired almost constantly. Tiredness is much more often of emotional origin and usually stems from boredom, frustration or an inability to achieve necessary standards. Many people with an overactive nervous system often develop feelings of exhaustion from time to time. Similarly, lassitude often becomes manifest when the normal hormonal balance is disturbed so that many women feel abnormally tired just before the period starts. Consequently, it is always difficult to say whether tiredness represents a metabolic or organic disorder as opposed to an emotional one. The tiredness of diabetes may become very profound. A young man may scarcely have the energy to get up in the mornings and may notice a falling off of strength in performing manual tasks. Associated with this tiredness is a general lack of zest and sex interest. Indeed, sexual impotence is not an uncommon cause for the patient to seek medical advice and for diabetes so to be discovered. In women, amenorrhoea, or cessation of the periods, frequently occurs in undiagnosed diabetes.

Many other minor symptoms may be noted on questioning in newly diagnosed diabetics. There may be a change in visual acuity. Patients often have to change their glasses because they note that their eyesight is blurred from time to time. These visual changes are not of serious connotation and are due to the presence of excess sugar in the fluid of the eye which temporarily alters refraction. When the blood sugar is restored to normal, these visual disturbances soon disappear. Another symptom is that of tingling in the fingers and feet. This too is a temporary phenomenon brought about by irritation of the nerves due to the excess sugar. Cramp in the calves and pain in the legs is a similar manifestation of excess sugar and can be sufficiently severe to wake the patient at night.

Especially in elderly women who are obese, perhaps the commonest presenting symptom of diabetes is that of pruritus vulvae, which means irritation of the genitalia caused by deposition of urinary sugar. This sets up disturbing itching and the scratching which resuts may cause infection with bacteria or fungus. Since this is not a symptom which women like to talk about, it is not uncommon for very severe inflammation and infection of the whole areas to occur before advice is sought. It can lead to a great deal of misery and discomfort with sleepless nights, though happily it is easily cured by appropriate treatment. This symptom is not restricted to the elderly and indeed it may occur in children or young women, and may be a presenting feature of diabetes. As with the other symptoms diabetes is not the only cause, though it certainly is the commonest of pruritus vulvae.

Before the discovery of insulin, diabetes was often associated with infection, and boils and carbuncles were very commonly present. It is customary today to test the urine for sugar in all cases presenting to the doctor with a boil or carbuncle though it must be said that these conditions are very common and are only occasionally associated with diabetes. Similarly, pulmonary tuberculosis used to be extremely common in diabetes since the weary, emaciated sufferer was very liable to pick up any infection and tuberculosis then was much more common than now. The combination of diabetes and consumption was a particularly lethal one, but happily today both conditions are treatable even when they occur together.

Diabetes sometimes presents to the doctor when the patient is in coma and this will be discussed later in more detail. Coma is much less common today than it used to be since most patients have the good sense to call on their doctors long before this state of affairs has been allowed to develop. It is always preceded by thirst, polyuria and loss of weight, but it can be very rapidly precipitated by an infection. Infection exacerbates the symptoms of diabetes and, particularly if associated with vomiting, soon leads to excessive production of acetone and so promotes the onset of coma. Any infection can produce this effect. A streptococcal infection of the throat, an infection of the ear, a patch of pneumonia, appendicitis, pyelitis (infection of the kidney) or phlebitis (infection of the veins), all have been known to precipitate diabetic coma. The symptoms of thirst and polyuria become more pronounced, the patient becomes so weary and weak that he can scarcely slake his thirst and the breathing becomes deep and laboured. When the patient has been admitted to hospital in coma he presents a striking picture. He is emaciated, his extremities are cold, the pulse is feeble and rapid, the blood pressure is low, the breathing is deep and sighing, and the breath smells of acetone. The diagnosis is confirmed by testing the blood for sugar and vigorous treatment must be instituted.

4

TABLETS FOR THE TREATMENT
OF DIABETES

TABLETS

In severe diabetes, there is no substitution for insulin. However, since 1955 tablets have been available for the treatment of mild diabetes developing in middle age. These tablets do not contain insulin and are not substitutes for insulin. They bring down the level of sugar in the blood to normal in mild diabetics and are consequently referred to as oral hypoglycaemic agents. This is regarded as a better term than anti-diabetic tablets since it does not imply that these tablets overcome all the features of diabetes. They merely reduce the raised blood sugar to normal.

HISTORICAL

In the late 1930s, the Germans produced a compound known as prontosil which had been found to be effective in destroying bacteria in the laboratory, and was equally efficacious when tried with patients. This was the first chemotherapeutic agent ever to be made available which could be safely taken by man to control bacterial infection. It overcame the effects of pneumonia and was astonishingly effective in reducing the ravages of various infections such as those which occurred after childbirth, the so-called post-puerperal infections. Unfortunately, prontosil itself was badly tolerated and made many patients feel desperately ill, even while it was overcoming the infection. Consequently, many other compounds of this type (known as sulphonamides) began to be produced which were equally efficacious in the treatment of bacterial infections but were less upsetting to the patient.

The search for more effective and better-tolerated sulphonamide compounds was continued in Germany after the war and in 1953 some new compounds, the sulphonylureas, were tried for the treatment of pneumonia in the wards of a Berlin hospital. Dr Fuchs, a young house doctor, noticed that some patients treated with one of these new preparations began to behave in an unexpected manner. Although the temperature had begun to fall and the signs of pneumonia were decreasing, the patients treated with this sulphonylurea began to sweat freely and behave in an irrational manner. Seeking for an explanation for this unexpected turn of events, Dr Fuchs wondered whether it could be due to a lowering of the blood sugar level, since hypoglycaemia (a low blood sugar) can produce these very symptoms. His suspicions were well founded. When the blood sugar was measured in these patients it was indeed found to be very reduced. He took the matter a step further by taking some of the tablets himself and was able to establish that they exerted a hypoglycaemic effect. There was lowering of his blood sugar and he developed symptoms of sweating and mental confusion. Since it now appeared established that these tablets exerted a hypoglycaemic effect, it seemed logical to try the effects in diabetics in whom the blood sugar levels were abnormally high. It soon became apparent that the sulphonylureas were no substitute for insulin in young diabetics, but in older and milder cases the elevated blood sugars could be restored to normal when the tablets were given.

Strangely enough, this was not the first demonstration that the sulphonylureas were effective hypoglycaemic agents. In 1942 a French physician, Dr Janbon, had been using similar compounds in Marseilles in the treatment of typhoid fever. He too observed hypoglycaemic effects and passed the compound to Professor Loubatieres working in Montpellier for further research. Professor Loubatieres, working with dogs and rabbits, soon confirmed that the tablets lowered blood sugar levels and he set about elucidating their mode of action. He was able to establish that these sulphonylurea compounds would only lower the blood sugar levels in dogs when the pancreas was intact. In dogs rendered diabetic by removal of the pancreas and so deprived of their source of insulin, no fall in blood sugar resulted when the sulphonylureas were administered. He deduced from these and other experiments that the sulphonylureas caused a reduction in blood sugar levels by stimulating the islet cells of the pancreas to produce more insulin. He was able to confirm his deductions by prolonged treatment with sulphonylureas in rabbits and demonstrated that the islet cells of the pancreas grew very much larger and produced much more insulin. Because of the circumstances then prevailing in France, Professor Loubatieres's work did not receive adequate recognition in medical circles and it was not until the clinical work of Fuchs that the importance of his investigations was realized.

Following the first clinical applications of the use of sulphonylureas, many compounds of this type have now been isolated and are in daily use in the treatment of diabetics. They all have the same broad effect in that they are only effective in mild diabetics in whom the pancreas is still capable of producing insulin under the influence of their stimulation. In young, severe diabetics the islet cells are incapable of producing any insulin whatever the stimulus and consequently the tablets are ineffective.

TYPES OF SULPHONYLUREAS

1. TOLBUTAMIDE

Tolbutamide was first introduced in 1955 and has proved to be a very safe and reliable tablet. It is a comparatively mild hypoglycaemic agent and its effect in reducing the blood sugar only lasts a few hours. Consequently it should be taken at least twice a day. It is very well tolerated which means that most patients can take it without feeling any ill effects whatsoever. Very rarely, an occasional patient complains of mild indigestion or develops a skin rash but this is quite exceptional. In mild diabetes, especially in elderly patients, tolbutamide will soon get rid of excess sugar in the blood and in the urine with relief of troublesome symptoms.

As with all the sulphonylureas, it will only be effective if the patient adheres to a diet. No tablet will be effective if the patient is overeating since the amount of insulin that can be produced under the stimulus of these tablets is strictly limited. The diet need not be of starvation level and usually will contain from 120 to 180 g of carbohydrate a day, quite adequate for most elderly people. Usually, within a week of starting the diet and the tablets, the patient begins to feel better and the sugar disappears from the urine.

The sulphonylureas can easily lead to an increase in weight. The increased output of insulin causes an increased conversion of carbohydrate to fat, another reason for the patient to be particularly careful about the diet. Increasing obesity is unhealthy, even though at the same time the blood sugar has returned to normal. Unless this tendency is watched very carefully, the mechanism for producing insulin soon breaks down and excess sugar returns.

The main disadvantages of tolbutamide are threefold. Firstly, it has to be taken two or three times a day because its length of action is short. Secondly, it is a comparatively gentle hypoglycaemic agent and not as effective as some of the newer compounds. Thirdly, and most important, many patients, initially well controlled when they take tolbutamide, begin to relapse after a variable time with return of sugar in the urine and diabetic symptoms. Sometimes this relapse is due to the fact that patients get careless about their diet and start to overeat again or to indulge in chocolates or biscuits. In many cases, however, the relapse is due to the fact that the islet cells of the pancreas are no longer able to respond and other treatment has to be substituted. This tendency to relapse is much commoner in patients with tolbutamide than with other compounds. The great advantage of tolbutamide is that it seldom causes the blood sugar to fall too low and so can safely be prescribed for elderly patients living on their own.

It should be realized that all these compounds are put on the market by various pharmaceutical firms who may not manufacture the compounds themselves. However, they will sell the compound under a name chosen by themselves. This means that any medical preparation may have more than one name. Tolbutamide is the official name for this particular compound but is marketed under various trade names, such as Rastinon or Pramidex, in this country. Nor are trade preparations of the same compound necessarily produced in the same form. They may be tablets of differing colour and shape or they may be in capsule form. This is often a source of confusion, particularly for cosmopolitan people who travel from one country to another. For this reason, most doctors prefer to use the official name (in this case tolbutamide) rather than the proprietary ones. Tolbutamide is produced in tablet form, each tablet containing 500 mg. The usual dose is one such tablet, two or three times a day, but as many as six tablets can be safely prescribed. In practice, if four tablets a day are ineffective, it is unlikely that a dose higher than this will make much difference in reducing the blood sugar. In a mild diabetic, a common starting dose is one tablet twice a day, at breakfast and at dinner. This can be increased to one three times a day if sugar persists in the urine.

2. CHLORPROPAMIDE

Chlorpropamide is a much more powerful hypoglycaemic agent than tolbutamide and its action in reducing blood sugar levels is maintained for more than 24 hours. Consequently, a single tablet given in the morning can keep the blood sugar down throughout the day. Furthermore, patients adequately controlled by chlorpropamide are much less liable to relapse with the passage of time than those treated with tolbutamide.

It suffers some disadvantages. Although it is well tolerated and completely safe for the vast majority of patients, occasionally it gives rise to drug rashes or even jaundice. Every drug carries with it a certain risk in that occasionally people react uniquely to some agents. Not everybody can take even coffee without untoward effects. Having said this, it should be added that chlorpropamide is an extremely safe preparation taken regularly by hundreds of thousands of diabetics. Its very effectiveness can be a disadvantage. In frail or elderly patients, the blood sugar levels can fall too low, especially at night time, with resulting confusion. This must be watched for carefully and the dose reduced when the blood sugars are restored to normal levels. On the whole, it is preferable to use tolbutamide in such patients.

Another unexpected effect of chlorpropamide is that it can react when alcohol is taken, giving rise to headaches and flushing. This is not usually troublesome, but patients taking chlorpropamide should be aware of this difficulty.

Chlorpropamide tablets are marketed in this country under the trade name of Diabinese and are in tablets of two strengths, one of 100 mg and a larger one of 250 mg. A usual starting dose is 250 mg each morning but some patients manage quite well on as little as 100 mg each morning, while others need 375 mg (one and a half 250 mg tablets). The dose should not exceed 500 mg daily since the risks of reactions increase above this dose level and the benefits of reducing blood sugars are not materially increased above 375 mg.

3. GLIBENCLAMIDE

Glibenclamide is another hypoglycaemic agent with a length of action similar to chlorpropamide but less likely to give rise to reactions when alcohol is taken. The starting dose is quite small. Usually one tablet (5 mg) taken in the morning with breakfast is sufficient to help control the blood sugar during the day. However, there is a good deal of variation and some patients may require as many as four tablets (20 mg). If taken in this way, it is usual to take some tablets at breakfast time and the others at lunch. In this way an even response is attained during the day.

Glibenclamide is available under two trade names, Daonil and Euglucon, each of 5 mg strength. These tablets are small in size, easy to take and do not upset the digestion. It is usual to start off with one tablet with breakfast in the morning, but in some patients this gives rise to too low a blood sugar level before lunch. In this case, the dose can be reduced to half a tablet. In others, as many as four tablets may be necessary to get rid of the sugar, but this dose should not be exceeded. In general, it can be said that if 20 mg is ineffective, there is no advantage to be gained by increasing the dose.

4. OTHER PREPARATIONS

Several other compounds are available and their action in the main is intermediary between those of tolbutamide and chlorpropamide. Such compounds are useful for patients who show idiosyncrasy or dislike for the compounds mentioned. Preparations at present available are set out in Table 4.1. It should be said that many physicians have learned to use one or other of these compounds regularly and, as there is not a lot to choose between them, the exact tablet that a patient receives is often a reflection of the particular experience of the doctor whose advice he seeks. It occasionally happens that a patient not feeling well on one type of sulphonylurea will improve on another, but it should be stressed that in the main the range of action of these tablets is very similar and no great benefit can be expected by transferring from one to another. Nor is there any advantage in adding another kind of sulphonylurea tablet to one already in use since they all act in the same way.

BIGUANIDES

As long ago as 1918, a German biochemist named Watanabe found that the compound guanide, which accumulates as a result of certain liver ailments, caused a lowering of blood sugar. Since at that time

TABLE 4.1   *The tablets*

Type	Official name	Proprietary name	Strength of tablet
Sulphonylureas	Acetohexamide	Dimelor	500 mg
	Chlorpropamide	Diabinese	100 mg
			250 mg
	Glibenclamide	Daouil	5 mg
		Euglucon	
	Glibornuride	Glutril	25 mg
	Glipizide	Glibenese	5 mg
	Tolazamide	Tolanase	100 mg
			250 mg
	Tolbutamide	Pramidex	500 mg
		Rastinon	
	Glymidine (a sulphapyrimidine)	Godafon	500 mg
Biguanides	Metformin	Glucophage	500 mg
			850 mg
	Phenformin	Dibotin	25 mg
			50 mg (capsule)

there was no effective treatment for diabetes, intensive research followed this discovery and culminated in the isolation of a group of compounds known as diguanides which were found to be effective in lowering the sugar in the blood when given by mouth in tablet form. Synthalin was one of these diguanides and was introduced by Franks for the treatment of diabetes in 1926. Although it reduced the raised blood sugar to normal in many diabetics, it was badly tolerated in that it gave rise to a feeling of sickness and often caused diarrhoea and vomiting. Furthermore, reports began to appear where jaundice had occurred in patients taking synthalin and this led to the belief that synthalin might have toxic effects on the liver. By 1926, insulin had become freely available and the need for synthalin was less pressing. Thus the drug fell into disrepute and disuse.

With the advent of the sulphonylureas in 1955, renewed interest was shown in the diguanides and by 1957 various compounds had been isolated in America by Ungar and in France by Sterne, which appeared to be both safe and effective. These compounds were derivatives of diguanides known as biguanides and in particular two preparations called phenformin and metformin became available for clinical trial in diabetic patients. These drugs were established as having no toxic effects on the liver and were completely harmless in this respect. They were highly effective in lowering the blood sugar but unfortunately were not always well tolerated. In many patients they gave rise to nausea, an unpleasant taste in the mouth and looseness of the bowel.

MODE OF ACTION

It soon became apparent that the biguanides reduced the blood sugar in a way entirely different from that of the sulphonylureas. The biguanides were effective even in animals in whom the pancreas had been surgically removed. This meant that they did not act by stimulating the islet cells of the pancreas to produce more insulin. Furthermore, although they were able to lower the blood sugar to normal when it was elevated in diabetes, the biguanides did not lower the blood sugar below the normal level as did the sulphonylureas.

Intensive investigation has so far failed to elucidate the exact way in which phenformin or metformin will reduce an elevated blood sugar level. At least three modes of action have been demonstrated. In the first place, it has been established that phenformin reduces the absorption of carbohydrates from the bowel. Phenformin often leads to a loss of weight and although this may be partly due to the fact that it reduces appetite, there is now convincing evidence that it causes a reduced absorption of food even when the intake is normal. However, it seems unlikely that this effect is sufficiently important to explain the profound fall in blood sugar levels that result when phenformin is taken. In the second place, experimental evidence has shown that phenformin reduces the amount of glucose produced by the liver. When there is a lack of insulin, the liver converts its stores of glycogen to glucose and glucose pours into the blood stream from the liver.

Phenformin inhibits this effect and so helps to keep the level of sugar in the blood nearer to normal. Thirdly, it has been demonstrated that phenformin encourages the muscles to take on more sugar. The muscles are deprived of glucose when insulin is deficient. When phenformin is administered, more sugar from the blood is able to enter the muscle and so provide metabolic fuel. It seems likely that the blood-sugar-lowering effect of phenformin is a summation of these three mechanisms. There is an impaired absorption of glucose by the bowel, a decreased output of glucose by the liver and an increased tendency for the muscles to use glucose. The net result is that less sugar circulates in the blood.

BIGUANIDE PREPARATIONS

Phenformin is the most effective biguanide preparation available for reducing blood sugar. It is available in two forms, tablets of 25 mg and capsules of 50 mg. The usual dose varies from 50 mg daily to 150 mg daily. A high proportion of patients, perhaps two-thirds, who take 150 mg of phenformin daily develop symptoms of gastrointestinal intolerance. They feel slightly sick, lose appetite, develop a metallic taste in the mouth and may even have bouts of vomiting and diarrhoea. When the dose is reduced to 100 mg daily, the blood-sugar-lowering effect is still significant and at this level only a small proportion of patients experience any unpleasant symptoms. Acceptability has been further improved by a capsule preparation in which phenformin is mixed with shellac. This delays absorption of the phenformin and considerably reduces the tendency to gastrointestinal ill effects. Most patients who take two capsules of 50 mg phenformin a day experience no ill effects whatsoever.

Metformin has a mode of action exactly similar to phenformin but its hypoglycaemic action is less effective. It is available in tablets of 500 and 850 mg and the usual daily dose is either three tablets of 500 mg or two tablets of 850 mg. On the whole, these tablets are less likely to give rise to gastrointestinal effects at this dose level, but they are not so effective as phenformin in reducing the blood sugar.

INDICATIONS FOR USE

As with the sulphonylureas, biguanides are most useful in middle-aged mild diabetics. Unlike the sulphonylureas, they tend to lead to a loss of weight rather than to an increase. They are therefore the drug of choice in mild diabetics who have a tendency to obesity since they not only reduce the blood sugar level but also help to keep down the weight. As with the sulphonylureas, they will only be effective if the patient is prepared to co-operate and to adhere to a restrictive diet, usually of the order of 1500 cal.

OTHER EFFECTS

It has been demonstrated that occasionally phenformin has been associated with a disorder known as lactic acidosis. Lactic acid is a by-product of the breakdown of carbohydrate and is usually excreted by the liver. Phenformin has the capacity to delay this removal of lactic acid and therefore lactic acid can accumulate in the blood. In ordinary circumstances, it is not important but if other ailments are also present which increase the lactic acid in the blood, the results can be disastrous. For example, in severe heart, lung or kidney disorders, an excess of lactic acid tends to form and, if the patient is concurrently taking phenformin, the lactic acid can rise to a level sufficiently high to lead to coma. Although this event is very rare, it means that phenformin should never be prescribed to patients who are not otherwise in good general health. Indeed, phenformin has now largely been replaced by metformin since, although severe lactic acidosis is a very rare complication in patient with phenformin, occasionally deaths have been reported. For this reason, metformin is now the biguanide of choice in this field since it does not give rise to this unfortunate complication.

COMBINED THERAPY

Since it has been established that the sulphonylureas and the biguanides have different modes of action, it is not surprising that they have an additive effect in reducing elevated blood sugars when given together. Thus, in patients who fail to respond satisfactorily to a sulphonylurea such as chlorpropamide, the addition of phenformin or metformin can often restore a normal blood sugar. As has been mentioned, many patients who respond initially to the sulphonylureas, tend to relapse after a variable length of time with a return of diabetic symptoms and the appearance of sugar in the urine. Here again, the addition of metformin will often clear up these symptoms and maintain a normal blood sugar without the need for insulin. It is safe to say that the use of combined therapy has enabled many moderately severe diabetics to maintain a normal blood sugar who would certainly otherwise have needed insulin. These patients may need both tablets of chlorpropamide and metformin taken together to keep the sugar in the blood at a normal level and the urine free from sugar.

CHOICE OF TABLET

When diabetes develops in adult life and when the symptoms are mild, many patients can be restored to normal health by a simple dietary restriction. A strict diet reduces the call for insulin and enables the reduced amount available to cope with the situation with restoration of the blood sugar to normal. If diet alone is barely effective, it is unreasonable to expect the patient to endure a starvation diet indefinitely. It is not only unreasonable to expect this, in practice few patients will tolerate too rigid a diet for any length of time. Since there is firm evidence that a raised blood sugar is ultimately detrimental to health, it is incumbent on the physician to prescribe oral hypoglycaemic agents. If the patient is of normal weight or even underweight, the sulphonylureas are the drugs of choice. They are safe and well-tolerated. In elderly patients tolbutamide can be prescribed; in younger ones a more effective agent such as chlorpropamide is preferable. If the patient is overweight, metformin may be the preparation of choice. Most people tolerate metformin very well, usually one tablet (500 mg) twice a day, and it helps to keep the weight down. If the patient fails to respond adequately to this, a combination of chlorpropamide or glibenclamide given with metformin is usually successful in restoring the blood sugar to normal. However, if the combination of these two tablets does not work, then injections of insulin must be substituted.

5

TREATMENT OF MILD DIABETES

~⟨§§§⟩~

DIAGNOSIS OF MILD DIABETES

The word mild in this context means that the blood sugar levels are not very much elevated above normal and so the condition does not give rise to troublesome symptoms. Indeed, as often as not there are no symptoms at all and the diagnosis is made by the chance finding of sugar in the urine. This may happen because the patient has been examined for a life insurance policy or because he has seen his family doctor and examination included a routine urine test. Mild diabetes usually comes on in middle age and is often diagnosed by chance in this sort of way. It must be stated, however, that although the term mild is true as far as symptoms are concerned, this form of diabetes can lead to considerable damage to the health of the patient unless it is adequately treated.

The diagnosis of diabetes cannot be made on a simple examination of the urine alone because sugar can appear in the urine even with a normal blood sugar, the condition known as a low renal threshold. Consequently, in order to confirm the diagnosis, a glucose tolerance test must be performed and this can conveniently be arranged at a local hospital. Normal unrestricted meals must be eaten for the three days preceding the test. The last meal should be taken on the evening before the test and the patient must arrive at the hospital without having had any breakfast or morning drink. After he has rested for half an hour, a blood sugar test is taken and he is given a drink containing 50 g of glucose. It is usual to draw blood for sugar estimation from the vein in the arm, a simple and relatively painless procedure.

After each half-hour further specimens of blood are taken, the last two hours after the initial drink, making five blood tests in all. If possible, urine is obtained at one hour and at two hours. The sugar in the blood and urine specimens are now estimated in the laboratory. If the fasting blood sugar exceeds 110 mg/100 ml, if the highest blood sugar after the glucose drink exceeds 180 mg/100 ml, or if the blood sugar at the end of two hours fails to fall below 120 mg/100 ml, then diabetes is present.

The confirmation that diabetes is present provides occasion for the doctor to make a full general examination of the patient and there are various points that will need to be checked carefully. The eyes will be examined, the blood pressure taken, the heart tested and the pulses felt both in the arms and in the feet. An X-ray of the chest is advisable and an electrocardiogram may be also necessary. Thus, the doctor can assess the general health of the patient and in particular, can determine whether or not the previously undiagnosed diabetes has done any harm. It will be understood that there is no precise onset to diabetes and the blood sugars may have been elevated for many months or even years before the diagnosis is established. It is generally taken that in mild diabetes there has been an elevation of the blood sugar level on average of eighteen months before symptoms begin to appear.

DANGERS OF MILD DIABETES

There is now substantial evidence that a raised blood sugar, in some ways like high blood pressure, can do damage in the long term. In particular, elevation of the blood sugar may be responsible in part for hardening of the arteries and a disposition to coronary thrombosis. Certainly, the incidence of arteriosclerosis and coronary thrombosis is very much higher in patients with an abnormal glucose tolerance curve than in people of the same age whose glucose tolerance curve is normal. It is also very likely that cataracts in the eyes and other complications occur more frequently when sugar is in excess. It is apparent that every effort should be made to restore the blood sugar levels to normal to preserve good health in the years ahead.

DIET

The most important aspect of the treatment of mild diabetes is to restrict the amount of food that is eaten. Although there may be a genetic tendency to diabetes, this is always exacerbated by over-eating which precipitates the onset of the ailment. The pancreas of a patient genetically disposed to diabetes is quite incapable of producing sufficient insulin to cope with excessive amounts of food. Perhaps this defect is a graded phenomenon. In other words, many people with a strong and healthy supply of insulin can manage to overeat without developing diabetes. On the other hand, if the pancreas has an inherent weakness excessive feeding soon causes it to break down.

The diet prescribed will depend on the weight of the patient in relation to the ideal weight for his height and age. The more obese the patient, the more restricted the diet will have to be. In a subject whose weight is 20% in excess of the ideal, a diet of 800 cal will be necessary. As will be seen in Chapter 12, this diet contains very little carbohydrate. The quality of the carbohydrate is just as important as the quantity. It must contain adequate dietary fibre. Wholemeal bread is better than white bread and the diet should contain plenty of salads, vegetables and fruit. Sugar and all foods containing sugar must be avoided completely, as must starchy foods such as biscuits, cakes and puddings. Protein is more satisfying and nutritious than carbohydrate and is available as meat, fish, chicken, eggs, cheese and milk. The vegetables contain very little food value but provide roughage and vitamins. In spring and summer, for example, salad and cheese provide an easy lunch. It is essential for the patient to provide himself with a weighing scale in the bathroom and to be weighed at the same time each day. Attempts to reduce weight can be a discouraging process and it must be realized that the weight tends to fluctuate day by day, sometimes according to whether the bowel or bladder has been recently emptied. Nevertheless, if an 800-cal diet is rigidly adhered to, it can be anticipated that the patient should lose 3 or 4 lb each week. It is worth stressing that the diet must be adhered to for seven days a week. Many patients follow the diet rigidly for most days but tend to have a 'blow-out' every now and again when they dine out. This is a temptation that must be resisted if the weight is to be reduced.

When the weight has been reduced to a level of 10% above the ideal weight, the diet can be increased to 1200 or 1500 cal daily. This allows more carbohydrate in the form of bread or potatoes and although restrictive it is not an intolerable diet for most people. Once again the measure of success is provided by the weighing scale and no amount of explanation and excuses can alter the simple fact that weight will be reduced if the patient is eating less than the body needs for energy purposes. Over and over again we hear obese people say that they cannot lose weight despite rigid dieting. They must be deluding themselves. It is a simple fact that since the body excretes material via the bladder and bowel and since fuel is constantly being used to provide energy for normal activities, then the reserve stores of fat must inevitably get smaller unless the food intake exceeds what is lost. It is perfectly true that some people seem to put on weight very easily and they need sympathy in this respect. But it remains undeniable that if the intake of food is reduced sufficiently, weight will be lost.

URINE TESTING

As a rule, the urine quickly becomes free from sugar when less food is eaten. In most mild diabetics, as soon as the intake of carbohydrate is restricted the strain on the pancreas is reduced and the insulin production becomes adequate to deal with the situation. Normal blood sugar levels are soon restored but the patient should not be lulled into a sense of false security when the sugar disappears from the urine. The gain may be only a temporary one. Unless the weight is brought down to a near normal level, inevitably the blood sugar will gradually start to rise again with return of sugar in the urine and subsequent danger to health. The best way of testing the urine in this type of diabetes is by use of Clinistix strips. These are plastic strips containing a small area of impregnated material at the tip. This is coloured light pink and provides an extremely sensitive test for sugar. In the presence of sugar, the pink colour turns darker and attains a purple tint. The speed at which the change of colour occurs and the depth of the colour is a rough guide to the amount of sugar but is too inaccurate to be useful in a quantitative respect. Its real advantage is that it gives a clearcut answer as to whether or not sugar is present. Since the blood sugar is likely to be at its highest level after lunch or after dinner, the best time to test the urine is in the mid-afternoon or in the evening in this type of diabetes. If the Clinistix test is negative at this time, then a repeat test once a week is adequate. The test should be repeated daily if sugar is present, and this fact must be reported to the doctor. As will be seen, persistent glycosuria (sugar in the urine) may be an indication for the introduction of tablet treatment.

ALCOHOL

Alcohol provides calories and as such can be regarded as a form of food. Consequently, it is best avoided altogether in the early stages when every effort is being made to reduce weight. Ultimately, when dieting has been successful in getting rid of surplus fat, alcohol can safely be taken in moderate quantities. There is no specific harm in alcohol, providing the weight is at a reasonable level and the urine free from sugar.

EXERCISE

There is no doubt that exercise helps to promote good health and every mild diabetic should take regular exercise providing the general examination reveals no serious contraindications. The amount and degree of exercise should be suitable to the patient's age and previous activities. The tendency to lead a legless existence is a thoroughly bad one. Too much time is spent in the armchair watching the television, in the chair at the office desk and in the car. The circulation becomes sluggish under these circumstances and disposes towards thrombosis or clotting in the arteries and veins. It pays to keep fit.

As to what form of exercise should be taken, this will vary according to circumstances. A skipping-rope, a rowing-machine or weightlifting exercises are perfectly suitable for use in the home, but there is nothing so good as a walk in the open or a game of golf. For those more active, squash or tennis is very effective but it is unwise to take up strenuous exercise over the age of 50 in somebody whose muscles have been inactive for many years. Taking the dog for a walk and gardening are beneficial and sufficiently energetic for most elderly people.

SMOKING

Smoking cigarettes is one of the most harmful habits of modern times. The medical profession is dismayed by the dreadful toll produced each year from lung cancer. But this is not the only disaster. Cigarette smoking strongly disposes to coronary thrombosis and since this is particularly liable to occur in diabetes, it is only commonsense for any diabetic to give up cigarettes entirely. Twenty cigarettes a day means over 7000 cigarettes a year. It can be seen that at this rate it takes less than thirty years to have smoked 200 000 cigarettes. This is probably a fairly critical level above which the dangers rapidly multiply. Cigarette smoking has a variable effect on individuals. Some people can smoke heavily all their lives and get away with it. Many are particularly sensitive to the evil effects and succumb in their early 50s. Attempts to cut down on cigarette smoking are nearly always useless, since inevitably the quantity smoked starts to creep up again. The only way to deal with cigarettes is to be convinced of their danger and to stop smoking forthwith. Happily, cigars and pipes seem to be far less harmful and are often a useful halfway measure in giving up the habit entirely. The tragedy is that many patients who have tried unsuccessfully to give up cigarette smoking do so overnight when they learn the dreaded fact that they have developed lung cancer. Too late, alas.

SUPERVISION

The patient with mild diabetes who has reduced his weight to a reasonable level and whose urine is consistently free from sugar still needs medical supervision from time to time. In the first place, it helps him not to be careless about his regime if he knows he has to see his doctor. In the second place, it is valuable to have a record of blood sugar levels, since the urine itself is not an entirely reliable guide to sugar in the blood. For these reasons, it is sensible for the mild diabetic to attend his doctor or the hospital clinic for advice and supervision every few months.

INDICATIONS FOR TABLETS

Despite careful adherence to the diet, in many mild diabetics the urine does not become completely free from sugar. Sometimes, although the urine shows very little sugar, the blood sugars are still elevated above normal. As there is growing evidence that excess sugar in the bloodstream is ultimately harmful, this is a situation that is best avoided. Under these circumstances, treatment with tablets becomes necessary. It is far better to take a tablet or two each day than to run the risk of ultimate deterioration of the health, though it is a pity to have to resort to tablets when the lack of success is merely due to the fact that the patient has not kept carefully enough to the diet.

When the doctor is faced with a patient who is failing to respond fully to simple dietary restriction, he will be guided as to what tablet to prescribe in part by the patient's weight and in part by his particular experience in this field. Mostly, if the patient is overweight, the doctor will tend to prescribe one of the biguanides since these tablets help to reduce weight while at the same time lowering the blood sugar. There is no question that the counsel of perfection for overweight patients is to get their weight down to a normal level, but if they seem unable to do this on simple dietary restrictions, then the biguanides are often successful in helping to achieve normal weight. Metformin is a biguanide and is given in the form of a tablet (500 mg) which can be taken before each main meal of the day. The majority of patients will tolerate this dose without any untoward effects but some develop a sense of nausea or looseness of the bowel sufficiently troublesome to make it unpleasant for them to continue at this dose level. In such cases, metformin can be given once or twice a day according to the effect required.

In patients of normal weight or those below normal, a sulphonylurea compound is usually prescribed. Tolbutamide is a very mild tablet and has to be given two or three times a day. It seldom causes the blood sugar to fall too low and is very useful in elderly patients in whom the attainment of complete normoglycaemia (a normal blood sugar) is seldom as important as in younger patients. It is well tolerated and hardly ever gives rise to troublesome effects. One tablet can be taken after breakfast and another after lunch. Chlorpropamide is a more effective hypoglycaemic agent than tolbutamide and need only be taken once a day after breakfast. Its effect in reducing blood sugar levels lasts all day and indeed can sometimes cause the blood sugar to fall too low during the night. For this reason, it is best not to use this tablet in the very elderly, particularly when they live on their own. As will be seen from Table 4.1, other similar types of compound are available with actions broadly similar to those of tolbutamide and chlorpropamide, the main difference being that of length of action. Every physician experienced in the treatment of diabetes will have gained experience in using one or other of these preparations regularly and will only need to change to a different compound if an individual patient is not responding well to the one first used. However, it should be stressed that if one of these preparations given in full dose is not successful in restoring normoglycaemia it is unlikely that an alternative sulphonylurea will do much better.

RISKS OF TABLET TREATMENT

Tablet treatment for diabetes has now been in use for over twenty years and the number of complications due to tablets is extremely small.

The biguanides sometimes give rise to gastric and intestinal upsets but these usually occur within the first few weeks of treatment, if at all Although this may make the patient feel unhappy and unwell, they do no permanent harm and the symptoms soon cease when the tablets are discontinued. Very occasionally, patients who have been taking the biguanides for several months begin to develop a sense of nausea and loss of well-being, feelings which disappear when the treatment is changed. More rarely still, phenformin or metformin can cause an increase of lactic acid in the body and this is particularly liable to occur when there is some other serious ailment at the same time, such as pneumonia or coronary thrombosis. The excess lactic acid causes the patient to feel drowsy and ill. For this reason, it is best not to use phenformin during any major illness. It may be wiser temporarily to substitute insulin even though the blood sugars have been quite normal.

The sulphonylureas scarcely ever give rise to trouble. Occasionally, patients complain of a feeling of fullness in the stomach or a mild sensation of sickness. Even less commonly, some patients react by developing a skin rash and if this happens it is wise to change the patient to a different compound. Jaundice very rarely occurs and when it does so, it is more likely to be due to a virus infection than to a reaction to the tablets. However, it is always wise to stop tablet treatment if jaundice appears just in case this might be the cause. Certainly, in the early days of treatment when large and excessive doses of tablets were used jaundice appeared from time to time suggesting a toxic effect on the liver.

It should be realized that the sulphonylureas can interact with other tablets or substances. One curious aspect of this is that chlorpropamide and alcohol when taken together lead to a flushing of the face and a sensation of throbbing in the head. This is not in any way dangerous but it is wise for patients taking chlorpropamide to realize that this reaction is liable to occur if they take an alcoholic drink. More importantly, many drugs taken for other purposes potentiate the action of the sulphonylureas and cause an excessive lowering of blood sugar levels. Some of the tranquillizers (the mono-amine oxidase inhibitors) react in this way with the sulphonylureas. To a lesser extent, so do aspirin and other tablets taken for relief of pain in the joints. Sufficient to say that any patient taking one of the sulphonylureas should be aware of the possible risks of taking other tablets at the same time.

The effect of lowering the blood sugar to too low a level (hypoglycaemia) is very much less marked in patients taking tablets than in those taking insulin. Hypoglycaemia never occurs with the biguanides and seldom occurs with the sulphonylureas. The fall in blood sugar caused by the sulphonylureas is gradual and usually allows time for other hormones to restore the sugar level to normal. In elderly patients, however, drowsiness, confusion, or even coma can occur when the blood sugar falls too low as a result of treatment with the sulphonylureas. In many patients, there is a sense of hunger, a tremulous sensation, a mild blurring of vision, a feeling that all is not well, all of which are most liable to occur some hours after the last meal was taken, or after unusual exercise. It seldom gives rise to any real trouble and offers no hazards to those driving a car. The usual cause of hypoglycaemia in patients taking tablets is that the dose is in excess of their needs. It should be realized that in the early stages of treatment with tablets a much larger dose is necessary than is ultimately needed once the blood sugar has been restored to normal. For example, a patient initially requiring 350 mg chlorpropamide (one large 250-mg tablet and one small 100-mg tablet) each morning to restore the blood sugar levels to normal will safely be able to reduce the dose after a month or so and may ultimately be quite well controlled on 200 mg (two 100-mg tablets) each morning. This reduction implies that the patient is keeping to his diet and is not allowing his weight to creep up. Indeed, one of the commonest causes of relapse or worsening of diabetes in patients taking tablets is that carelessness in diet has occurred and the patient has begun to eat more than he ought. The keystone of the successful treatment of mild diabetes is adherence to the diet and maintenance of a steady weight.

The diet of patients taking tablets should be a reasonable one that can be kept to regularly without the patient constantly feeling hungry. In practice, this means a diet varying from 1500 to 2000 cal according to the patient's age, size and activity. A careful check must be kept on the weight and, although initially every effort must be made to reduce excess fat by rigid restriction, once a satisfactory weight has been reached, food intake can gradually be increased providing the urine and blood tests are satisfactory and providing the weight is not increasing. The urine must be tested regularly with Clinistix. Initially, it is best to test the urine each day after lunch until it is seen that the urine is regularly sugar-free. Thereafter, testing the urine once a week is adequate providing no sugar is present.

RELAPSE

Unfortunately, many patients who are well controlled initially with tablet treatment may start to relapse after a few years with return of glycosuria (sugar in the urine) and symptoms of diabetes. Although this is often due to the fact that the patients have become careless about the diet, in many cases relapse occurs for other reasons. Since diabetes tends to be a progressive ailment, in some patients the supply of insulin from the pancreas becomes less and less and ultimately, despite stimulation by sulphonylureas, the output of insulin fails altogether. For this reason, it is important for all diabetics taking tablets to test the urine regularly and to attend their doctor or clinic at regular intervals, so that the first sign of trouble can be detected and appropriate measures adopted.

TREATMENT OF RELAPSE

If there is any suggestion that the relapse is due to dietary indiscretion, then a tightening of the regime in this respect will often be enough. However, if the patient and doctor are both confident that this is not the case, then treatment with combined tablets becomes necessary. This means that the patient now takes both sulphonylureas and biguanides together. For example, a patient who has begun to relapse on 350 mg of chlorpropamide a day, can now also take 500 mg of metformin twice a day in addition. Since these two compounds act in different ways, the combination is often successful in restoring normoglycaemia where either compound on its own was unsuccessful. Indeed, some physicians prefer to start treatment in new diabetics with both compounds straight away where they feel the diabetes is moderately severe and unlikely to respond to either tablet separately.

However, if a combination of tablets is unsuccessful, it is no use persisting with diabetes uncontrolled. This will only lead to the dangers of infection and other complications in the long run and it is much better to start on insulin. Many patients who have resisted the idea of insulin and persevered too long with tablets, feel so much better in themselves when they start on insulin that they regard the inconveniences of injection as a minor disadvantage.

PRINCIPLES OF GOOD HEALTH FOR
THE MIDDLE–AGED DIABETIC
(See Chapter 12 for details of diet)

1. Avoid sugar, syrup, honey, jams, chocolates, sweets, cakes, biscuits, puddings and all starchy foods: they are bad for you.

2. Avoid too much fried foods, fat and cream.

3. Eat plenty of fresh fruit of all kinds, vegetables and salads.

4. Eat lean meat, chicken, fish, cheese and eggs.

5. Eat wholemeal bread rather than white bread, and take All-Bran or other high fibre cereals especially if the bowels are constipated.

6. Keep your weight down to a level which is appropriate for your age and height. Cut down on food intake, especially carbohydrate, if the weight is not satisfactory.

7. Take regular exercise suitable for your age: use your legs.

8. Do not smoke in any shape or form but above all avoid cigarettes.

9. Have a regular check of the urine and blood to make sure you are not making too much sugar.

10. Enjoy yourself. There is no reason why you should not keep healthy and enjoy a ripe old age if you look after yourself: diabetes in middle age is not a serious disorder if properly managed.

6

INSULIN

~§§§~

HISTORICAL

Diabetes is an ailment with such striking and characteristic features, especially when developing in young people, that it is not surprising that it was recognized as a disease entity even in ancient times. Indeed, it has been claimed that the Papyrus Ebers, which dates approximately from 1500 B.C., contains a reference to diabetes mellitus and a prescription for treatment. Perhaps the best of the ancient descriptions is that by Aretaeus the Cappadocian who wrote in Greek in the second century A.D. A translation of his work states:

Diabetes is a wonderful affection, being a melting down of the flesh and limbs into urine. The patients never stop making water, the flow is incessant, as if from the opening of aqueducts. The patient is shortlived if the constitution of the disease be completely established; for the melting is rapid, the death speedy. Moreover, life is disgusting and painful; thirst unquenchable; and one cannot stop them either from drinking or making water. Their mouth becomes parched and their body dry; the viscera seem as if scorched up and at no distant term they expire.

References to diabetes continued from time to time but no great advance in the understanding of the complaint was reached until Thomas Willis discovered that the urine of diabetics was sweet. In 1679, he wrote:

The urine of the sick is so wonderfully sweet, or hath an honeyed taste; the urine is deprived of its salt taste but why that it is wonderfully sweet like sugar or honey, this difficulty is worthy of explanation. As to what belongs to the cure, it seems a most hard thing in this disease to draw propositions to curing, for that its cause lies so deeply hid and hath its origin so deep and remote.

In 1775, Dobson recognized that the sweet material in diabetic urine, which Willis had detected by tasting the urine, was indeed sugar. In the early part of the nineteenth century improving techniques in biochemical analysis enabled the sugar to be identified as glucose. Further studies by Bernard revealed that not only was there excess sugar in the urine but, more important, the sugar in the blood was also elevated above normal levels. In a series of brilliant experiments on dogs, he deduced that the excess sugar in the blood was produced by the liver. Indeed, as we know today, in uncontrolled diabetes excess sugar is produced by the liver from its stores of glycogen. But this defect is secondary to the lack of insulin.

The knowledge that the pancreas played the primary role in the cause of diabetes arose from a chance finding by Minkowsky. This physiologist had set out to determine the role the pancreas played in the digestion of food. It was known that the pancreas produced digestive enzymes which were excreted into the bowel via a duct and Minkowsky decided on an investigation as to what happened to the digestion of food in the bowel when deprived of the pancreatic juices. To this end he embarked on the operation of removing the pancreas from a dog, a new experimental procedure which demanded a high degree of surgical skill. The operation was successful but when he came to examine the animal the following day, to his surprise it had become piteously thirsty and was passing large quantities of urine which attracted abnormal numbers of flies. Minkowsky deduced and confirmed that the urine contained sugar, and soon was able to prove by measuring the sugar in the blood that the animal had developed diabetes. This work was reported in 1889 and caused a sensation in medical circles. It was the first time that any association had been established between diabetes and the pancreas.

The structure of the pancreas had long been the subject of exhaustive study and in 1867 Langerhans had already reported on the discovery of islets of cells quite different in structure from those which produced the enzymes. With the new knowledge that removal of the pancreas led to diabetes, the suggestion was made that the islets of Langerhans might contain a hormone, the absence of which would allow the sugar in the blood to accumulate.

The concept of hormones was well established by the turn of the century and already one type of hormone deficiency was being successfully treated. Patients suffering from a deficiency of the thyroid gland became sluggish and bloated. This was due to lack of thyroxin, a hormone secreted by the thyroid gland which controls body metabolism. This condition, known as myxoedema, had been successfully treated by the administration of extracts obtained from the thyroid glands of sheep and cattle. Hence vigorous attempts were made to treat diabetic patients in a similar way with pancreatic glands obtained from animals. Extracts obtained from mincing the glands were given by mouth or injected under the skin but led to no improvement of the diabetes or reduction of the sugar.

It is salutory at this point to look back at the treatment of diabetes in young people at the turn of the century. Once the diagnosis was made, the outlook was grave indeed and death usually followed within a few months or a few years at most. The only treatment which was in any way successful was that of almost complete starvation. Children were placed on a meagre diet of some 400 cal. It was argued that as the body was producing excessive quantities of sugar, it was unwise to give carbohydrate foods which could only exacerbate further this plethora of sugar in the blood. The guiding rule was that the less food that could be eaten the longer life could be sustained. The sabbath day was often made a day of complete starvation. It was difficult to admit these wretched children to hospital since they stole the food from other children's plates. There are pathetic accounts of children who ate their own toothpaste or who stole the birdseed from the canary cage. Despite these draconian measures, the end was inevitable. Slowly the flesh wasted, the breath became heavy with acetone and the child became more drowsy, until, perhaps mercifully, coma ensued from which no recovery was possible. Such was the background that acted as a spur to the desperate efforts to find a cure and was so stimulated by Minkowsky's discovery of the vital but enigmatic role of the pancreas.

Frederick Banting was a young Canadian surgeon who had served with distinction in the First World War and had returned to his native country to undertake a surgical post in Toronto. His interest in diabetes had been stimulated long before he took up medicine because the son of a neighbour had developed and died of this complaint. On his return from Europe, Banting had read an article in a medical journal giving the details of experiments on the pancreas which instantly aroused his interest. In these experiments, the pancreatic duct had been tied and when the pancreas was re-examined at a later date, the experimenter had found that all the enzyme-producing cells had degenerated, leaving the islet cells of Langerhans plump and intact. Banting felt sure that the islet cells contained the elusive hormone implicated in diabetes. He hit on the hypothesis that previous attempts to obtain effective extracts had been frustrated because the hormone from the islet cells had been destroyed by the enzymes also present in the pancreas when extracts were obtained from the untreated gland. This new technique of tying the duct and destroying the enzyme-producing cells offered the opportunity of obtaining the hormone undisturbed by enzymes. With this idea in his mind he approached Professor MacLeod of Toronto University in the spring of 1921 for permission to conduct experiments on dogs on these lines. Since Banting himself was not equipped to pursue biochemical studies, he was joined by Best, a graduate student selected by Professor MacLeod to help Banting measure the sugar in the urine and blood. Working with a small number of animals, Banting and Best tied off the pancreatic ducts and reopened the animals after ten weeks. They then removed the pancreas glands and confirmed under the microscope that the enzyme cells had indeed degenerated while the islet cells remained intact. They now obtained an extract by mincing up these glands and injected it into a dog rendered diabetic by the removal of the pancreas. The sugar level in the blood of this dog was very high and the animal showed symptoms of thirst and profound weakness. Within hours of the injection of their new extract, the dog became lively and active. Estimations of sugar in the blood showed that it had fallen precipitously following the injection and indeed had been restored almost to normal.

The new hormone formed in the islet cells of the pancreas was named insulin and the first human being ever to receive it was a 14-year-old diabetic named Leonard Thompson on 11 January, 1922. He was soon followed by six other patients and in all of them the insulin injections led to a dramatic improvement in their sense of well-being and a reduction of sugar in the urine and blood. This discovery led to worldwide interest and enthusiasm, and the names of Banting and Best will forever hold a hallowed place in the annals of medicine. Thirsty, emaciated, dying diabetics crossed the Atlantic from Europe to receive the new cure and Banting needed the co-operation of the most brilliant biochemists in Canada and America to work out more practical methods of obtaining insulin on a large scale.

PREPARATION OF INSULIN

The commercial production of insulin is now a highly organized operation. Soon after Banting's original procedure, it became apparent that it was unnecessary to destroy the enzyme-producing cells of the pancreas in order to obtain insulin from the islet cells. Further investigation revealed that if the glands were frozen immediately after removal from the animal, the operation of enzymes was completely inhibited and so extraction of insulin could be undertaken without damage.

Under modern commercial conditions, the frozen glands are obtained from cattle and pigs, arriving in sackloads from as far afield as the Argentine. The glands are ground in large grinding machines in the frozen state and are then placed in stainless steel extraction tanks containing acid alcohol. This method extracts insulin from the glands while suppressing the destructive activity of the enzymes present. The extract now contains insulin in alcoholic solution and the alcohol is next removed by high vacuum evaporators. What is left is largely insulin but in an impure state. Further technical processes are undertaken until the insulin is sufficiently cleared of impurities to be ready for human use.

Insulin has not only got to be pure; it also has to be standardized as to its potency. The standards are based on the degree to which the blood sugar is lowered in the rabbit following an injection of a measured amount of insulin. A dry stable form of insulin has to be prepared for these estimations and the standards necessary must be accurately followed by the manufacturers of insulin. Hence all forms of insulin now available have undergone stringent tests as to purity and potency before they are issued for use in diabetics.

Nevertheless, until recently most commercial insulins have contained traces of material other than insulin itself, especially pro-insulin. Pro-insulin is an inert molecule from which insulin is formed in the islet cells and some of it is released with insulin itself. It is very doubtful whether pro-insulin causes any material ill effects but insulins have been prepared without pro-insulin. This highly purified insulin is known sometimes as mono-component insulin, because it contains no components other than insulin itself. Mono-component insulins are more difficult to prepare and so are more expensive than insulins hitherto used.

STRUCTURE AND SOURCE OF INSULIN

The human pancreas is an elongated organ lying at the back of the abdominal cavity below the liver. It is comprised of two types of cells, the acinar cells and the islet cells. The acinar cells are those which produce the digestive enzymes and these cells are arranged in groups round a central opening. Each of these openings connects to small channels which ultimately join a main duct. The acinar cells thus ultimately excrete their digestive enzymes into the main pancreatic duct which leads into the duodenum, a part of the small intestine. As we have seen, these digestive enzymes help to break up proteins and fats which enter the small intestine from the stomach and so play a vital part in the digestive system. The second important structure of the pancreas comprises the islets of Langerhans. These are clumps of cells completely different in appearance from the acinar cells and not in any way connected to the system of ducts.

A great deal of study of these cells has been undertaken since Langerhans's original description. It is now realized that the islets contain at least two different types of cell and in some species as many as four different types of cell have been identified. The two most important cells that have been differentiated are known as the alpha and beta cells. When these cells are stained with certain dyes, it can be seen that they are of different structures. We are now confident that it the beta cells which produce insulin while the alpha cells produce glucagon, a hormone which appears to have a diametrically opposite effect to that of insulin. Where insulin reduces the sugar in the blood, glucagon tends to elevate it. In some species, for example in the duck and in the snake, the islet cells are composed entirely of alpha cells. In these creatures no insulin is produced at

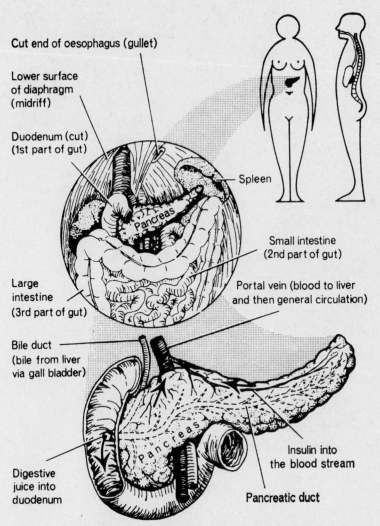

Cut end of oesophagus (gullet)

Lower surface
of diaphragm
(midriff)

Duodenum (cut)
(1st part of gut)

Spleen

Pancreas

Small intestine
(2nd part of gut)

Large
intestine
(3rd part of gut)

Portal vein (blood to liver
and then general circulation)

Bile duct
(bile from liver
via gall bladder)

Pancreas

Insulin into
the blood stream

Digestive
juice into
duodenum

Pancreatic duct

FIG. 6.1. In this diagram the stomach has been removed to show the position
of the pancreas in relation to the main organs
(Courtesy of Family Doctor Publications and Audrey Besterman)

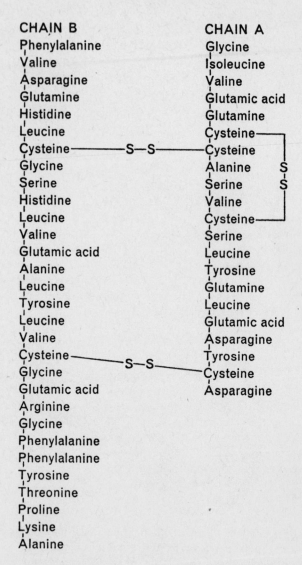

FIG. 6.2. The structure of insulin, containing 51 amino-acids

all and removal of the pancreas leads not to a rise in blood sugar but a fall in blood sugar following deprivation of glucagon. The part played by glucagon in man is somewhat enigmatic and probably not of great importance. Indeed, evidence has been produced that glucagon actually stimulates the production of insulin but the complexities of this situation are currently under investigation.

Until recently, investigation of the structure of the islet cells depended on the use of various types of stains which coloured different cells in different ways and so could be differentiated when examined under the microscope. In recent years, a new dimension has been added to our knowledge of the structure of the islet cells by the introduction of the electron microscope. This apparatus utilizes the short wavelength of an electron beam and has enabled the structure of the beta cells to be studied in molecular detail. We are beginning to get a clearer idea of how the insulin granules are formed in the beta cells and how they are released into the bloodstream. There are many factors which are seen to stimulate the formation and release of insulin granules. The most potent of these is a rise of sugar in the blood though how this stimulus is applied to the beta cells is quite unknown. Similarly, the sulphonylureas cause an increased formation of insulin. The insulin granules in the beta cells can be seen to be increased in size and number following prolonged administration of these compounds.

A puzzling feature of the structure of the pancreas is the fact that the islet cells are scattered in clumps throughout the substance of the gland, the majority of which consists of acinar cells. No other organ which produces hormones is similarly constructed, and there seems no valid reason why the islet cells should not have been concentrated together in a single organ, just as all the thyroxine-producing cells form a single organ, the thyroid gland. It has been suggested that the hormones produced by the islet cells, insulin and glucagon, may in some way nourish or influence the acinar cells and their proximity to the acinar cells allows actual passage of these hormones into the acinar cells. But this is at present speculation unsupported by firm evidence.

The structure of insulin has been completely elucidated by Sanger in 1955 when working at Cambridge, a work of such fundamental importance that he was awarded the Nobel prize. Sanger showed that insulin is composed of two chains of amino-acids bound together by two sulphide links. Altogether insulin is composed of 51 amino-acids. It will be remembered that amino-acids are themselves derived from the breakdown of proteins in the bowel and in the liver, and these amino-acids then become available for building up into various tissues of the body, including the hormones. Although commercial insulin is obtained from cattle and pigs, its biological effect in man is the same as human insulin. However, animal insulin is not identical in structure with that of human insulin. For example, bovine insulin contains three amino-acids which are different from those in human insulin. Three amino-acids out of 51 may seem a very small and unimportant difference but in fact this difference, though slight, is detectable by the human body.

In 1967, Steiner in Chicago was able to demonstrate that insulin is formed in the islet cells from a bigger molecule, which is called pro-insulin, and that some pro-insulin was released from the islet cells together with insulin itself. Pro-insulin is an inactive molecule and has no effect on the blood sugar.

Any foreign material which enters the human body causes a reaction. Thus when bacteria or viruses invade the bloodstream they provoke the formation of special proteins which block the effect of the invader. The foreign invader is called an antigen and the blocking proteins are antibodies. When we consider how many different types of bacteria alone can enter the system, it is an extraordinary fact that each different antigen will promote the formation of a specific antibody to counteract it. Since bovine and porcine insulins are foreign materials not identical with human insulin, their effect is antigenic and appropriate antibodies began to form. Unless highly purified, commercial insulins also contain pro-insulin and this too provokes antibody formation. In most cases, these antibodies are not sufficiently strong to block the effect of insulin to any material extent. In some patients, however, antibody formation may be sufficient partially to overcome the effect of insulin and so necessitate the injection of very high quantities of insulin to overcome this effect. This is known as insulin resistance. Happily it is not a very common phenomenon. Bovine insulin is much more antigenic than porcine and as most commercial preparations contain a mixture of bovine and porcine insulins in variable quantities, in recent years pure porcine insulin has had to be made commercially available. This insulin could prove of value in patients who become resistant to mixtures of bovine and porcine insulin or who show allergic reactions when ordinary insulin is injected. Furthermore, the artificial build-up or synthesis of insulin from its component amino-acids has already been successfully undertaken by investigators in the laboratory, so that it may be in years to come, synthetic insulin will be available without antigenic properties.

Insulin has to be injected under the skin or into the blood in order to be effective. It cannot be given by mouth because it is destroyed by the intestinal enzymes before it can be absorbed. Clearly, the disadvantages of injecting insulin would make it highly desirable to obtain a form of insulin which could be taken in tablet form but so far all attempts have failed. Ingenious methods have been tried such as enclosing insulin in a container which could be attached to the inside of the mouth and which would allow insulin to be slowly absorbed from the mouth without being swallowed. It certainly has been demonstrated that insulin is absorbed in this way but since the method is cumbersome and absorption unreliable the idea has not proved of practical value. At present, nothing can replace the need to inject insulin in patients whose islet cells are incapable of producing natural insulin.

TYPES OF INSULIN AVAILABLE

The first insulin used in diabetic patients is known as regular or soluble insulin and is a clear aqueous solution of insulin containing minute quantities of zinc to stabilize it. This form of insulin may be injected subcutaneously under the skin, into the muscle or directly into a vein. It is the only preparation of insulin which can be given intravenously, and is the only insulin available for emergencies such as diabetic coma. It exerts its effect very quickly in that it starts to remove excess sugar from the blood within an hour of injection under the skin and even more quickly if given into the vein. Its main disadvantage is that its length of action is short so that it will only keep the blood sugar level low for about 4–6 hours. At the end of this time the sugar in the blood starts to rise again and another injection must be given. In practice, therefore, in order to control the raised blood sugar in diabetes, soluble insulin must be given two or three times a day. Despite this objection, soluble insulin has a very useful part to play in the treatment of diabetes because its effect is reliable and injections can be given before breakfast and before the evening meal. Many physicians believe that this is the best form of insulin treatment for children, during pregnancy, or when there is infection present. In diabetic coma, very large quantities of soluble insulin must be injected in order to restore the blood sugar to normal and to get rid of the ketones which also form in the blood. The soluble insulin in this situation is given in part into the vein and in part under the skin. The intravenous insulin acts very quickly while the subcutaneous insulin acts more slowly but maintains its effect longer so that using both routes holds a definite advantage in a serious case where the patients is comatose.

Soluble insulin is prepared commercially in four different strengths. The weakest contains only 20 units of insulin for each millilitre of solution. This is usually written as 20 units/ml. This insulin is scarcely ever used since in order to give a usual dose of insulin, large quantities of this dilute solution need to be injected. It is useful in occasional patients who are unusually sensitive to insulin and require only a small dose to stabilize them. Nowadays, most patients who previously had to be controlled with a small amount of insulin are managed by tablet treatment, so there is very little call for insulin of this strength. The most usual strengths of insulin are either 40 units/ml or 80 units/ml. Since 1 ml is quite a large amount to inject, on the whole the 40-strength insulin is best reserved for patients needing 30 units or less for each injection. The 40-strength insulin can be measured more accurately than the 80-strength insulin because the amounts are larger and this is an advantage in elderly patients with poor eyesight. The 80-strength insulin is best used when the patient needs more than 30 units for each injection since the amount of solution to be injected to have the same effect is only half that of the 40-strength insulin. 40-strength insulin is sometimes referred to as double strength insulin when 20-strength insulin was regarded as the standard strength. There is no doubt that this is a most misleading description and often leads to confusion with patients receiving half or twice the required dose. In this country there is common agreement that 40-strength insulin is always in a container with a blue label while 80-strength insulin has a green label. A specially concentrated insulin has been prepared which contains 320 units/ml. This highly potent insulin is necessary in those patients who become very resistant to the effects of insulin, probably because they form antibodies to insulin. In such exceptional circumstances, patients may need some 600 units or more of insulin each day and the 320-strength insulin means that the amount to be injected is not unreasonably large.

There is a move afoot to replace the present 20-strength, 40-strength and 80-strength insulins by a single new 100-strength insulin and trials are being conducted to ascertain whether this should be introduced nationally. Of course this would entail a new type syringe with a narrower bore and markings to 100 for a 1-ml syringe. This new strength insulin and new syringe would do much to reduce the risks of confusing different strengths of insulin as is liable to happen at present. Even small quantities of this concentrated insulin should be easy to draw up accurately so long as the syringe has a narrow bore and the markings are clear and easy to read: but it must be admitted that small errors in drawing up insulin would lead to significant differences in the amount of insulin injected.

Two pure forms of soluble insulin are now available, prepared entirely from porcine insulin and freed from pro-insulin. These insulins are from Denmark and are called actrapid (Novo) and neutral (Leo Nordisk). They are less acid than soluble insulin and less antigenic.

TABLE 6.1   *Some insulin preparations*

Preparation	Source	*Antigenicity	Type of action	Maximum effect
Soluble	Beef	Moderate		
Actrapid	Pig	Very low	Short	2–4
Neutral	Pig	Very low		hours
Lente	Beef/Pig	Moderate		
Isophane	Beef/Pig	Moderate		
Rapitard	Beef/Pig	Low	Medium	4–12
Retard	Pig	Very low		hours
Zinc protamine	Beef	Moderate		
Ultratard	Beef	Low	Long	6–18
Monotard	Pork	Very low		hours

* Antigenicity means the capacity to provoke antibodies. Pork is less antigenic than beef insulin. Highly purified insulins have very low antigenicity.

They can be given directly into the blood (intravenously) just as ordinary soluble insulin.

ZINC PROTAMINE INSULIN

The fact that soluble insulin has to be given at least twice a day can be a real disadvantage to many diabetics who lead an active life and are away from home throughout the day. Consequently, following the discovery of soluble insulin, numerous attempts were made to prolong its action so that only one injection each morning would keep the blood sugar down to normal throughout the day. Attempts to delay the action of insulin by mixing it with oil were unsuccessful and it was not until 1936 that Hagerdorn in Denmark finally succeeded in producing a long-acting insulin which maintained its effect of reducing excess sugar in the blood stream for over twenty-four hours. He managed to modify the action of insulin by adding a type of protein known as protamine obtained from the sperm of certain fish. The resulting complex of protamine and insulin was made stable by the addition of zinc chloride to produce a milky solution. This form of insulin is slow to reduce the blood sugar and indeed may take six or eight hours to have any marked effect. To offset this disadvantage, it continues to exert its hypoglycaemic action for over twenty-four hours. In practice, zinc protamine insulin is not a successful method of controlling diabetes when given on its own since it is difficult to correlate the waning effect on the blood sugar of the injection given the previous morning with the delay in effect of the injection on the day it is given. However, zinc protamine insulin has proved extremely successful when combined with soluble insulin in a mixture. If soluble insulin is combined with zinc protamine insulin in equal proportions, there is sufficient free protamine to combine with the soluble and the resulting mixture is no different in effect from zinc protamine insulin itself. However, if two or three times as much soluble insulin is added to zinc protamine insulin, there is sufficient free soluble insulin to exert an immediate effect and sufficient zinc protamine insulin to maintain good control for the rest of the day. Thus a patient needing 60 units of insulin a day could be controlled either by an injection of soluble 32 units before breakfast and soluble 28 units before the evening meal, or by a single injection of a mixture containing 40 units of soluble insulin and 20 units zinc protamine insulin given once a day before breakfast in the morning. There is a good deal of controversy as to which method is the better. There is evidence that over the long term, soluble insulin twice a day offers better protection against the complications of diabetes and for this reason it is still preferred by many physicians as the method of treatment in children. In older patients the convenience of the single daily injection outweighs the possible dangers of ultimate troubles, perhaps not liable to occur for twenty or thirty years.

Many other forms of insulin have been made available since Hagerdorn's original discovery and although these have marginally refined the control of diabetes, it has made the choice of insulin unnecessarily confusing.

LENTE INSULIN

Lente insulin is a form of insulin in which insulin and zinc form a turbid suspension together without the addition of either protamine or globin. The precise action of zinc in modifying the action of insulin had not been fully investigated but in 1951 Hallas-Moller found that if the concentration of zinc was increased and the type of solution somewhat changed, a form of insulin could be produced with an extended length of action. This insulin could be purified in two different forms one crystalline and the other amorphous, the resulting solutions having different lengths of action. Lente insulin is available in three forms, semi-lente, lente and ultra-lente insulin, all of them differing in the duration of their activity. Semi-lente insulin acts quickly but exerts its effect only for a few hours. It is very like soluble insulin. Lente insulin itself has an intermediate length of action, while ultra-lente insulin is more akin to zinc protamine insulin. Although the lente insulins contain insulin uncomplicated by the addition of any other protein, in practice they have no real advantage over the preparations already mentioned. Lente insulin is usually prescribed for patients requiring less than 40 units per day, and its action can be modified by the addition of semi-lente or ultra-lente to suit the particular needs of the patient. Purer forms of these insulins are available and are called semitard, lentard and ultratard. They are more expensive but will ultimately replace semi-lente, lente and ultralente.

ISOPHANE INSULIN (NPH)

This insulin has an intermediate action similar to lente insulin. It is a cloudy solution containing protamine, as does zinc protamine insulin, but it acts much more quickly and its duration of effect is about twenty-four hours. It has one major advantage in that when it is mixed with soluble insulin each insulin retains its own individual action. Thus a mixture of soluble and isophane insulin permits the immediate though short-lived effect of the soluble insulin and the prolonged effect of the isophane insulin to be exerted independently. In patients requiring two injections of insulin a day and who are not well controlled by soluble insulin alone, the addition of isophane insulin to the morning injection can improve control without further incommoding the patient.

RETARD (LEO) INSULIN

Insulin obtained from pigs is slightly different from that of cattle and porcine insulin is more like human insulin than bovine insulin. Porcine insulin is therefore less antigenic. Retard insulin is similar in action and properties to isophane insulin but it is pure porcine and it has been freed from pro-insulin. It is a suspension of tiny crystals of insulin and its maximum effect is between 4 and 12 hours. It can be mixed with neutral (Leo) insulin which then covers the time before retard acts.

RAPITARD INSULIN

Rapitard insulin is also freed from pro-insulin and is a suspension of beef insulin crystals in porcine actrapid insulin. Its length of action and purity means that it is very like retard insulin. It can be mixed with actrapid if a quicker effect is needed.

7

TREATMENT WITH INSULIN

As has been described in a previous chapter, a large percentage of patients with diabetes can now be restored to normal blood sugars by watching their diet and taking appropriate tablets, without recourse to insulin. Nevertheless, there remains a type of diabetes which cannot be controlled without insulin. This is true of almost all cases of diabetes developing in children and in young adults. However, it is not only young diabetics who must be controlled with insulin and it is a mistake to assume that when diabetes develops in an older age it can necessarily be managed without insulin. Indeed, sometimes very elderly patients develop severe diabetes which does not respond to tablets and which cannot be controlled without insulin. In the main, patients who are underweight are unlikely to be controlled without insulin as are patients who show considerable acetone as well as sugar in the urine. The presence of acetone suggests a more serious derangement of metabolism and this is unlikely to be corrected by tablet treatment. Indeed, considerable amounts of acetone in the urine is perhaps the single most important indication for the need for insulin.

In the case of children and young adults, many physicians start off with insulin as soon as the diagnosis is made because the chances that they can be stabilized on tablets is rather remote. It is true that some young adults can be controlled for a time by a restricted diet and tablets. Unfortunately, the majority of these young people ultimately need insulin, since usually after a year or so the tablets lose their effect. Indeed, it is problematical whether it is worth starting with tablets in this type of patient when ultimately the chances are that insulin will be needed. At present, the state of our knowledge is not sufficiently precise in this direction to be dogmatic and each case has to be judged on its merit by the doctor in charge.

An important indication for insulin is when the tablets fail in their purpose of keeping down excess sugar from the bloodstream and from the urine. Tablets are not lucky charms and if they are not being successful in maintaining normoglycaemia (normal blood sugar) then insulin should be substituted. It must be understood that there is little point in taking tablets when the blood sugars are not controlled. In such cases, insulin is necessary since only in this way can the blood sugars be restored to normal once tablets become ineffective. Tablet treatment can only be regarded as justifiable when the blood sugars are kept normal and the patient is feeling well.

Insulin often becomes necessary when a patient with diabetes develops an infection. It is not known why infection causes a deterioration in diabetes, but it nearly always does so. Tonsillitis, an attack of bronchitis or pneumonia, an infection in the kidney, or inflammation of the veins are examples of ailments which cause a temporary deterioration in diabetes. Patients previously well controlled on tablets may temporarily need insulin under these circumstances, though once the infection has been suitably treated, very often tablets can be reinstituted and insulin discontinued. Similarly, sometimes the patient taking tablets for diabetes may need temporary insulin if he undergoes a major operation and the diabetes temporarily becomes out of control.

Naturally, insulin is always necessary in any severe case of diabetes when coma is threatened or when the onset is precipitated by a serious illness. Insulin is the only effective way of restoring normoglycaemia and ridding the blood of ketones under these circumstances.

INSULIN ROUTINE

Once the necessity for insulin has been established, the sooner the patient learns how to inject himself, the better. He may well be instructed to inject himself from the first injection so that he can gain confidence in his ability to look after himself. Instruction is often given while the patient is in hospital but sometimes instruction can be given in the doctor's consulting room, so long as the patient has sufficient confidence to manager further injections on his own.

The choice of which insulin to use is decided partly by the age of the patient and by the severity of the condition, and partly by the doctor's particular preference. As has been stated earlier, there are a variety of insulins available and there is no such thing as the best insulin. Each case will be decided on its merits. In the main, patients needing large amounts of insulin may require two injections a day, usually given half an hour before breakfast and half an hour before the evening meal. Patients who are controlled by a small dose of insulin are usually stabilized on a single injection of a long acting insulin given before breakfast. When a patient is admitted to hospital for initiation of treatment, he may be given soluble insulin two or three times a day until the blood sugars are restored to normal and the urine becomes free from sugar. If this happens quickly and the total dose of insulin is only 30–40 units a day, then a single injection each morning will be enough.

INSULIN ONCE A DAY

Some diabetics, particularly elderly people, do not need a large amount of insulin, perhaps because they still produce some insulin of their own. In such cases, the diabetic can be controlled by an injection of insulin each morning, given half an hour before breakfast. The insulin given can either be an injection of a simple intermediate insulin, or as a mixture of two insulins given in the same syringe.

There are many different types of intermediate insulin (see Table 6.1) suitable for a single daily injection because they continue to be absorbed gradually during the day. Lente, isophane, retard and rapitard are all effective insulins in this situation: but it must be stressed that their activity is beginning to wear off overnight. Hence, a mixture of a short with medium or long acting insulins are often advised since each insulin retains its individual effect. For example, soluble insulin can be mixed with isophane insulin in the same syringe. Broadly speaking, the soluble insulin keeps the blood sugar down in the morning (when the blood sugar is mostly likely to be raised), and the isophane insulin covers the rest of the day and overnight.

INSULIN TWICE A DAY

When good control of the diabetes is important, particularly in children and young adults, or where the insulin requirements exceed 40 units a day, insulin is best given twice a day, before breakfast and before the evening meal. The insulins used are usually a short acting insulin (soluble, neutral or actrapid) to which is added in the same syringe an intermediate insulin (isophane, retard or rapitard). In this way good control of the blood sugar can be maintained throughout the day.

The combinations which work well together include soluble and isophane; neutral and retard; and actrapid and rapitard.

Assuming a mixture of neutral and retard is being taken, the first injection should be given before breakfast. The neutral covers the morning; the retard covers the afternoon. The second injection is given before the evening meal. This neutral now controls the blood sugar before bedtime and the retard comes on to work overnight (see Fig. 7.1).

INJECTION ROUTINE

Special syringes are available for the injection of insulin and since 1954, there has been a British Standard insulin syringe, known as BS1619, available under the National Health Service for insulin injections. It is a glass syringe with metal fittings, and is available in two sizes, the smaller of 1 ml and the larger of 2 ml capacity. Each millilitre is divided into 20 marks, which means that the numbers on the syringe are easy to read even for patients with poor eyesight. If the patient is using insulin of 40 units/ml strength, than each mark on the syringe contains 2 units. A patient needing 36 units of this strength insulin will draw up to the 18 mark on the syringe. If the 80-strength insulin is used, then each mark is worth 4 units. In this case, a patient needing 36 units will draw up to the 9 mark.

The syringe can be kept in a spirit-proof case made of aluminimum, designed to immerse the syringe in industrial methylated spirit to reduce the risk of bacterial infection. There is really no need to boil the syringe frequently as was thought to be necessary in the past. Needles for injection are of various sizes and perhaps the most suitable is the 26 GX¼", which is sufficiently fine to make the injection relatively painless. The needles too should be kept in industrial spirit and it is often best to have a separate needle for drawing up the insulin, since the fine point of the syringe may be blunted when pushed through the

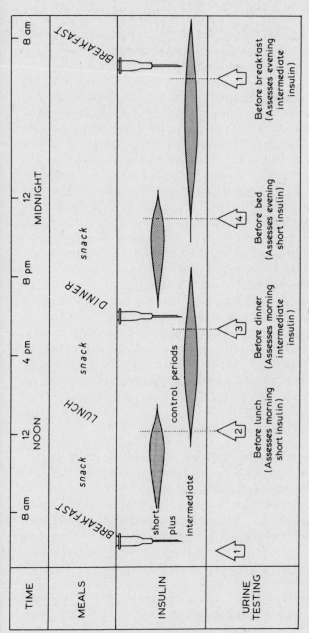

FIG. 7.1

Notes

1. Snacks are taken mid-morning, tea time and before bed.
2. Suitable short and intermediate mixtures are:

   Soluble plus isophane; neutral plus retard; actrapid plus rapitard
3. The proportions of short and intermediate and the amounts can be assessed by the appropriate urine tests; e.g. if the before-lunch tests always show a lot of sugar, increase the morning short insulin; if there is a tendency to reactions overnight, reduce the evening intermediate insulin.

rubber cap of the insulin bottle. Usually, with care, a needle can be used for many injections without losing its sharpness.

Disposable syringes are now available for insulin injections, some with a needle attached. These plastic syringes have been sterilized in their sealed containers by gamma ray radiation, which destroys all bacteria without the need to heat the syringe or to add spirit. These disposable syringes are extremely convenient, particularly when on holiday. The only snag is that of expense since disposable syringes are not obtained on prescription under the NHS unless in exceptional circumstances through a hospital consultant. Disposable needles are also available and these too can be obtained through the NHS at the discretion of the hospital doctor. These needles tend to be sharper than non-disposable ones and can be safely kept in spirit. Disposable needles are suitable for use with the ordinary glass and metal syringes and can be used for at least a week. Although it is not advised by the manufacturers that a disposable syringe and needle should be used for more than one injection, in practice some patients use the same disposable syringe and needle for a few days at a time without running into trouble. Nevertheless, the counsel of perfection is to use a fresh disposable syringe and needle for each injection. It must be stressed in this respect that disposable syringes are available for many purposes other than the injection of insulin and care must be taken that the BS1619 type disposable insulin syringe is requested and obtained.

SITE OF INJECTION

Insulin is best injected subcutaneously, that is to say, under the skin. It is painful and inadvisable to inject into the skin itself since this causes local swelling. A fold of skin can be lifted with the thumb and finger of the left hand and the needle pushed firmly into the fold below the skin itself (see Fig. 7.2). The needle should be injected at an angle of 75° so that the insulin is injected into the loose fatty tissues lying under the skin. Patients sometimes fear that they may accidentally inject into a vein. In practice, this fear is groundless and indeed would be quite harmless even if it occurred.

The usual sites of injection are the outer side of the thigh, the lower part of the abdomen or in the upper arm (see Fig. 7.3). Most people find the outer side of the thigh the simplest and most convenient. It is best not to use exactly the same area each time, since this leads to

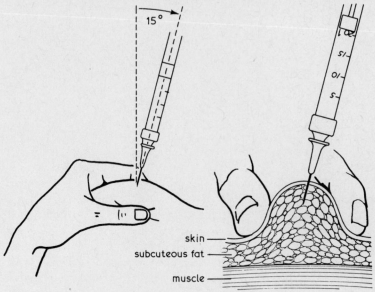

FIG. 7.2. A simple method of injecting insulin

toughening of the skin and soreness. A different area should be chosen each day and both legs can be alternated, the right leg on even calender days, the left on the odd.

Two injection aids are available and are sometimes helpful in the early stages of insulin injections in children or nervous adults. The Hypoguard Automatic Injector consists of two parts, a needle holder which is attached to the syringe and a needle guard which is placed in position over the needle when the syringe has been filled to the appropriate level with insulin. Sharp pressure on the body of the syringe springs the needle through the skin and the insulin is then injected in the usual manner. The Palmer Injection Gun is a holder for the filled syringe and attached needle. Pressure on the trigger fires the needle through the skin and allows the insulin to be injected as usual by pressure on the plunger. Both apparatuses relieve the onus of actually pushing the needle through the skin, though in practice most people soon overcome this compunction and the apparatus is discarded.

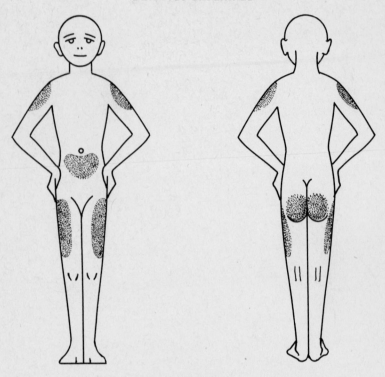

FIG. 7.3

DRAWING UP THE INSULIN

Once the syringe and needle have been assembled it is best to draw back the plunger before pushing the needle firmly through the cap of the insulin bottle. The insulin bottle can be left to hang on the needle which is quite strong enough to take this weight. Both hands are now free, one to hold the syringe and the other to work the plunger. The plunger should be pushed upwards, thus forcing air into the insulin bottle. This means that the insulin in the bottle is under slight pressure and draws more smoothly into the syringe when the plunger is withdrawn to the required level. The insulin in the syringe must be carefully inspected to see whether any air is present. If a bubble of air is seen the plunger must be pushed upwards again and then drawn back to the required level. The syringe and needle should now be withdrawn from the bottle and a new needle inserted for injecting under the skin. Ordinary washing is all that is necessary as far as the hands are concerned, but the area of skin to be injected should be cleaned with lint dipped in spirit. Disposable swabs soaked in spirit and sealed in foil are also available at most chemists. It is quite exceptional for infection to occur if commonsense and a routine of ordinary cleanliness is observed.

In mixing two insulins together, the following routine should be followed (see Fig. 7.4):

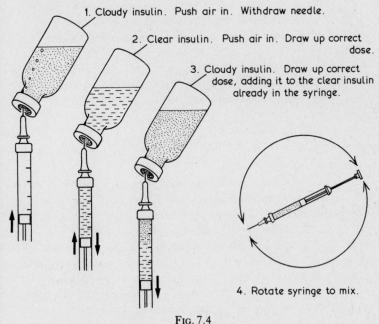

1. Cloudy insulin. Push air in. Withdraw needle.

2. Clear insulin. Push air in. Draw up correct dose.

3. Cloudy insulin. Draw up correct dose, adding it to the clear insulin already in the syringe.

4. Rotate syringe to mix.

FIG. 7.4

(i)   After cleansing the top of each bottle with spirit, push some air from the syringe into the cloudy (intermediate or long acting) insulin bottle.

(ii) Withdraw the needle and push some air into the clear (short acting) insulin bottle.

(iii) Draw up the clear insulin to the required mark and withdraw the needle.

(iv) Draw up insulin from the cloudy bottle to the required level adding it to the clear insulin already in the syringe. Since air has already been pushed in, the insulin in this cloudy bottle is under pressure and so easier to withdraw.

(v) Rotate the syringe once or twice to mix the two insulins ready for injection.

Thus if a patient needs 32 units of soluble insulin plus 16 units of isophane insulin, he will first draw up into the BS1619 syringe 8 marks of 80 strength clear insulin from the soluble insulin bottle and then 4 marks of cloudy insulin from the isophane bottle, making a total of 12 marks on the syringe and containing 48 units of the mixture. One or two rotations of the syringe are sufficient to give a uniform mixture of the two insulins before injection.

Insulin bottles should be kept in a cool place. The refrigerator is quite satisfactory, but not the freezer compartment. Insulin loses its potency after a time and should not be used after the date stated on the bottle.

LOCAL DIFFICULTIES OF INSULIN INJECTIONS

1. ALLERGY

Since insulin is derived from non-human sources, it is not exactly the same as human insulin and so may give rise to local allergic reaction at the site of injection. The area of injection becomes red, swollen and itchy. This phenomenon is nearly always restricted to the first few weeks of insulin injections, presumably because the patient ultimately becomes desensitized to this effect. As a rule, the allergic reactions are not sufficiently severe to occasion much distress, particularly if the patient understands that it is only a temporary disturbance. It can be partially prevented by taking anti-histamine tablets, though these sometimes give rise to some drowsiness. These allergic reactions seldom occur with the purified porcine insulins, such as actrapid or retard, and it is worth changing over to one of these insulins if the older type of insulin was being used.

2. LIPODYSTROPHY

This is a troublesome condition, occurring almost entirely in women, in which the subcutaneous fat at the site of the insulin injection tends to atrophy or waste and gives rise to unsightly pits. This is not in any sense a serious condition in that it causes no general disturbance, but it can be disfiguring if the hollows are extensive and if they occur in areas liable to be noticeable when wearing a bathing costume. The real cause of this dystrophy is not known. It was suspected that it might be due to contamination of the insulin with industrial spirit but no evidence has shown this to be so. The fact that it occurs in women and not in men may partly be due to the fact that women have more subcutaneous fat in the thighs than men but a more likely explanation is that there may be some female hormone which reacts with the insulin locally and then causes dissolution of the fat.

It is often advised that the best way of avoiding these pits is to change the site of insulin injection as frequently as possible so that no one particular area is always receiving injections. Although this advice may be helpful, it must be confessed that it is not always successful in preventing lipodystrophy from occurring. Strangely enough, perhaps the best way of causing the pits to fill out is to inject the insulin directly into the pit itself, preferably using one of the purer mono-component insulins.

3. LIPOHYPERTROPHY

In some patients, sometimes in men, exactly the opposite to lipodystrophy occurs. Instead of fat dissolving at the injection site, it tends to increase and give rise to humps or mounds at the site of injection. These are usually less troublesome than the atrophic pits and are not usually unsightly. Here again, the cause of this disorder is unknown and perhaps the best way of avoiding this trouble is to vary the site of injection each day.

4. LOCAL INFECTION

Providing the syringe and needles are kept in spirit and ordinary cleanliness is used when injections are given, local infection should not occur. It is quite exceptional for an abscess to form at the site of an injection because the insulin is sterile and is too acid to form a good medium for bacteria to grow.

URINE TESTING

Diabetic patients needing insulin injections are well advised to test the urine regularly, particularly if the urine tends to show sugar from time to time. It is often unwise to attempt to have all specimens of urine free from sugar since this may carry with it the risk of hypoglycaemic reactions. Some mild diabetics find that the urine is always sugar free on a single injection of insulin each morning, but it is commoner to find variable degrees of sugar in the water from time to time. The most useful times to test the urine are in the early morning, before lunch, before the evening meal and last thing at night. In each case it is more instructive to test urine that has not been lying in the bladder for many hours. Thus, it is best to empty the bladder on waking in the morning, and then to pass another specimen for testing just before breakfast. This will give a good indication of the level of the fasting blood sugar. Similarly, the bladder should be emptied at about 11 a.m. and another specimen obtained for testing just before lunch. The bladder can be emptied at about 10 p.m. and then the final specimen passed for testing just before going to bed. Whereas in patients taking tablets the urine should be free from sugar, in insulin diabetics this is not always attainable. A simple Clinistix test is usually not adequate in this case since it does not define the amount of sugar present. Consequently, it is best for most insulin dependent diabetics to test the urine with Clinitest tablets, since this gives a useful estimation of how much sugar is present in a quantitative way. A newer strip test called Diastix is now available and may be equally reliable. After immersion in urine for two seconds, the colour change of the strip must be compared with the chart on the bottle after exactly 30 seconds. When sugar is present, the colour changes from green to varying degrees of brown. A chart should be kept setting out the day-to-day results of urine testing since this gives the doctor a useful guide as to progress and whether insulin or diet need adjustment.

BLOOD TESTING

There is now available a simple method of estimating the amount of sugar in the blood and one which the diabetic can learn to do for himself. The pulp of the thumb is stabbed by a stylet (available in sterile packets) and a blob of blood placed evenly across the prepared end of a Dextrostix strip. Exactly one minute later, the blood is washed off the strip by a jet of water and the area dried. The depth of colour (which varies from light mauve for a very low blood sugar to deep purple for a high blood sugar) can now be compared against the colour chart on the Dextrostix bottle containing the strips, giving a rough idea of the level of blood sugar. However, a more accurate measure can be made by placing the Dextrostix into a Reflectance Meter, a photoelectric apparatus which allows a quantitative reading to be made. The method is simple and quick and relatively painless, and is reliable if the instructions are carefully followed. Unfortunately, the Reflectance Meter is expensive. The great advantage of the method is that it allows the diabetic to get a clearer idea during an ordinary working day of what the blood sugars are standing at. This means that the insulin dose can be adjusted more accurately than from a knowledge of the urine tests alone.

8

DIET AND CONTROL
OF DIABETES

〜✧✧✧✧〜

Many patients who develop diabetes are alarmed initially at the thought of keeping to a diet for the rest of their days. They seem to forget that the word diet does not imply anything more than a restriction on overeating, and that they can continue to eat and enjoy good food in the future as they have done in the past. No diabetic today who takes insulin need go hungry or thirsty. The key to success is an understanding of the principles of diet and the value of the particular articles of food that are eaten. Every diabetic should understand clearly the carbohydrate, protein and fat content of food and should understand the make-up of the meal he is eating. The diet should be nourishing and appetizing, and should be so balanced that it contains adequate quantities not only of carbohydrate, protein and fat but also of vitamins, minerals and roughage. In devising a diet, many factors must be borne in mind. The previous eating habits of the patient are the basis of the diet. Although various diet sheets can be provided which suit the majority of people living in this country, any dietary regime which attempts to impose a radical revolution in the eating habits of a particular patient is doomed to failure. The modern dietitian will always make careful inquiries as to the patient's normal eating habits and will only adjust these habits if they are unsuitable to the diabetic situation. No use attempting to impose a diet of bread and potatoes on an Indian lady who has eaten rice and curry all her days, and who will certainly go on doing so if an attempt is made to impose a diet altogether alien to her habits and inclinations.

The amount of carbohydrate, protein and fat to be taken will vary both as regards the total amount and as regards the proportions of each type of food according to the age, size and activity of the person in question. Investigations of the general population have demonstrated a surprising variation from person to person in the amount of food that is eaten, often apparently bearing little relation to activity or weight. It must be accepted that appetite is a variable factor and some people can eat more than others without putting on weight. Consequently, although a diet may be chosen initially which seems about right for the age, weight and activity of the patient concerned, adjustment will have to be made in the light of experience. A careful watch will have to be kept on the weight which must be kept as near normal as possible. Obesity goes badly with diabetes. Of course, in the early stages of diabetes, the patient may well be considerably under weight and the diet will have to be ample enough to allow the patient to reach a more normal size. Once an ideal weight has been achieved, the diet can be cut back to some extent. Appetite is an important factor. Some patients complain that the diet is more than they can manage and more than they have eaten in the past. Others may complain that they are hungry all the time. In either case, adjustments can be made.

Once the amount of food has been decided, the next question is what proportions of carbohydrate, protein and fat should be eaten. It can be said that there is no unanimity of opinion as to what is the ideal make-up of the diet in this respect.

Fat is the most concentrated form of food, yielding 9 cal for each gramme, more than twice that of either carbohydrate or protein. Unfortunately, large amounts of fat are not palatable. There is another more cogent reason for a diet high in fat to be undesirable in that fat may be a precursor of substances which cause arteriosclerosis or hardening of the arteries. This is a controversial subject. It is generally agreed that an association exists between the level of cholesterol in the blood and a tendency to coronary thrombosis. It is also agreed that cholesterol may be derived especially from certain types of animal fats. What is in doubt is whether a life-long restriction of fat intake will successfully reduce cholesterol and so reduce the incidence of coronary thrombosis and arteriosclerosis. Intensive research is proceeding into this subject at the present time. It has been demonstrated that not all types of fat give rise to an increased level of cholesterol. Animal fats are particularly prone to do so but certain vegetable oils (comprising the so-called polyunsaturated fatty acids) may actually

reduce cholesterol levels, at least temporarily. For this reason diets
have been promulgated in which all animal fats (including butter) are
replaced by fats from such sources as corn oil and the vegetable oils.
These diets are expensive, tedious, and unappetizing. The benefits
are dubious, and in the present state of our uncertain knowledge,
most doctors will hesitate to impose this regime unless special circumstances dictate its necessity. In the main, the diabetic diet should not
contain excessive quantities of fat and the amount prescribed is
usually sufficient to make up the calorie content of the diet when adequate quantities of protein and carbohydrate have been prescribed.

Protein is a valuable but expensive form of food and there is no
reason for the diabetic diet to contain more or less than that normally
eaten. Indeed, many doctors place no particular stress on the amount
of protein, leaving it to the patient's individual taste. In adults, a re-
commended minimum of 1 g of protein daily for each kilogramme of
ideal body weight is regarded as satisfactory. In practice, this means
about 75–85 g of protein a day. Proportionately larger quantities will
be needed in children and during pregnancy.

Carbohydrate is the food that is most important to regulate in diabetes. In the early days it was felt that since sugar is obtained from
carbohydrate, the less carbohydrate eaten the better. Further experience showed that this thesis was erroneous since in fact it merely led to
an increased breakdown of fat and a consequent increase in production of dangerous ketones. Consequently, it is now generally
agreed that the diabetic taking insulin must have a minimum of 180 g
of carbohydrate a day and as much as 300 g may be necessary for a
young man doing very heavy work.

Once the patient has grasped the essentials of diet he can be given
an outline diet sufficient for his needs. All forms of carbohydrate foods
are interchangeable, so that, for example, bread can be substituted for
potatoes, and rice substituted for either. The amount of fibre in these
foods must be borne in mind, since refined foods are more quickly
digested and broken down to sugar than carbohydrates containing a
high content of dietary fibre. Wholemeal bread is better than white
bread and brown rice preferable to polished rice. Potatoes should be
eaten in their jackets. All-Bran, Shredded Wheat and porridge oats
are preferable to Corn Flakes or Rice Krispies. Fresh fruit, raw vegetables and salads contain dietary fibre and vitamins though they do

not have a high carbohydrate content.

When he has learned the calorie value and fibre content of the common articles of carbohydrate food and knows how much he is allowed for each meal, he can eat with freedom wherever he happens to be. Similarly, protein foods and fats can be altered according to needs. A meal of meat and potatoes can easily be substituted for one of cheese and bread, since both contain measurable quantities of protein and carbohydrate.

In patients taking insulin it is of paramount importance that mealtimes should be regular and the food regularly spaced throughout the day. In non-diabetics, if a large meal is eaten, large quantities of insulin are produced in response to the sugar absorbed from the bowel. If no food is eaten, no insulin is produced. This subtle mechanism is lost in the diabetic requiring insulin. The insulin injected in the morning goes on exerting its effect irrespective of whether food is eaten or not. Consequently, if the insulin is injected and no food eaten, the sugar in the blood becomes too low and may give rise to hypoglycaemic reactions. It is therefore of paramount importance for every diabetic taking insulin to ensure that he eats regular meals at regular times and that he never gets caught out by being late for a meal. Indeed, as will be elaborated later, he must always carry sugar with him and take it at the first sign of a hypoglycaemic reaction.

It is fair to say that once a diabetic taking insulin has grasped the basic principles of diet he will find no real difficulty in eating out, going abroad or camping, since he can adjust the amount he eats to suit his requirements. The diet should be one of regularity and discretion but not of restriction and prohibition.

Some diabetics never lose their sweet tooth and it is possible for them to take artificial sweetening agents in this respect. Cyclamates have gained a bad reputation, probably unjustifiably, and have now been prohibited. However, saccharine is safe and inexpensive. It has no food value whatsoever and is passed unchanged in the urine. It has a sweetening taste and can safely be taken in beverages or in cooked food. In some people, it leaves a somewhat unpleasant aftertaste but in most it is indistinguishable from sugar. Another sweetening agent is sorbitol. Sorbitol, a derivative of alcohol, is a form of food which has a calorie value similar to that of sugar but does not cause an elevation of sugar in the blood. Consequently, unlike sugar itself, it can be taken without noticeably increasing blood sugar levels. It has a mild laxative effect, especially if taken in large quantities and since it has a calorie value, it should be taken in moderation. Many diabetic foods contain sorbitol and it can be used as a sweetening agent in chocolates, biscuits and jam. Proprietary foods purporting to be suitable for diabetics merely replace sugar by sorbitol, fructose or saccharine. They tend to be expensive and are neither as wholesome or satisfying as natural foods.

Since all carbohydrate food is ultimately broken down to glucose or other monosaccharides in the bowel, it may be asked why sugar itself should not be taken. The answer is that sugar is a highly concentrated and unnatural form of carbohydrate, very rapidly absorbed from the bowel and imposing considerable stress on the storage mechanism. It tends to cause a too rapid rise of sugar in the blood and this in turn calls for an increased demand for insulin. The breakdown of ordinary carbohydrate foods such as bread or potatoes is much more gradual, formation and absorption of glucose is slower and much less likely to lead to a rapid change in blood sugar levels. Hence, for most insulin-dependent diabetics food containing sugar or glucose is best avoided.

Alcohol may be taken in discretion by diabetics on insulin, providing the diabetes is stable and there is no tendency to frequent hypoglycaemic reactions. Alcohol is a form of food and has a calorie content, higher in the sweeter drinks (which contain sugar) than in the drier varieties, so that this must be allowed for in estimating the calorie intake. In patients liable to reactions, alcohol may further confuse the issue and it has been known for a diabetic in a hypoglycaemic reaction to be mistaken for a drunk because the breath smelt of alcohol, a potentially very dangerous error.

EXERCISE

Just as it is important for the diabetic taking insulin to avoid obesity and to keep to a regular diet, so it is important for the young diabetic to keep fit and active. The muscles need exercise to prevent the circulation becoming too sluggish. There is no doubt that activity reduces the propensity for the blood sugars to rise though unfortunately it has become increasingly difficult to keep fit in modern life. Most occupations today are sedentary, much of our leisure time is spent in front of the television and most of us live so far away from work that we have to travel by transport rather than use our legs. This means that many young people only take adequate exercise if they set out deliberately to do so. It is particularly important for the young diabetic on insulin to keep fit and there is really no restriction on the type of exercise that can be taken. Simply going for a walk each day is a good start but a more positive attempt to take exercise should be encouraged, perhaps by playing such games as tennis or golf. Skating, bowling, skipping, squash, or even dancing are all exercises suitable for the young diabetic. Swimming is an excellent pastime though it offers the risk of hypoglycaemic reactions while in the water. It is best not to swim out of depth and to avoid swimming before mealtimes. It should be stressed that bursts of violent activity may reduce the blood sugar too rapidly and this danger must be appreciated, so that it is wise to take sweetened drink before any intensive exercise. In general, it pays to take regular exercise, to use the legs and not to allow the circulation to become too sluggish.

ADJUSTMENT OF INSULIN

Every diabetic taking insulin should test the urine and record the results as a guide to progress. In the main, if the urine shows persistent significant quantities of sugar in the urine, it may be necessary to increase the dose of insulin without seeking the advice of the doctor on every occasion. Usually, the increase of insulin can be in the order of 10–20 % when glycosuria (sugar in the urine) has persisted for more than a few days. It must be realized that there are natural variations in the level of blood sugars, probably unconnected either with the diet or with the insulin. Many diabetic patients are puzzled by the fluctuations that occur in urinary sugars and usually try to relate such fluctuations to the meals they have eaten the previous day. Of course, it is true that if an unusually heavy meal has been eaten, there is much more likely to be an increased glycosuria the next day. However, excess food is not the only factor which will cause increased glycosuria. There are several hormones apart from insulin which can affect blood sugar levels and these are under the control neither of the diet nor of the insulin injected. Also, the amount of exercise taken varies from day to day and this affects the amount of sugar used up by the body. Furthermore, although the potency of insulin is carefully standardized it may not always be absorbed at the same rate. If the injection is made into a particularly hard area below the skin, the insulin may be poorly absorbed. Another cause of variation in urinary sugar is that of infection. Even mild infections such as a common cold or a sore throat can temporarily increase the need for insulin and so lead to an excessive glycosuria. Consequently, the diabetic taking insulin must not feel guilty or apprehensive if the urine starts to show more sugar than usual. In many diabetics fluctuation of this sort is inevitable, however careful the dietary and insulin regime, and even if the amount of exercise taken is the same every day. It is most unwise to be constantly altering the insulin dose in response to occasional increases in urinary sugar. This merely leads to uneasiness and insecurity and does not necessarily lead to improved control. However, if urinary sugar is persistently increased for several days, it is as well to temporarily increase the insulin. It can always be lowered to the previous level once the situation has righted itself. Equally important, if the urine is constantly free from sugar and if reactions begin to occur, it may be necessary to reduce the insulin dosage. There is no doubt that the less the patient has to alter the insulin dose the better, and the doctor will always be able to advise if the urinary sugars and blood sugar tests are unsatisfactory. He will be able to assess from the pattern of the urinary tests whether adjustment of the amount or type of insulin has become advisable.

CONTROL OF DIABETES

Good control of diabetes implies relief of symptoms and the maintenance of a fit and healthy life. There is evidence that a blood sugar constantly elevated at too high a level disposes to poor health in later life and for this reason doctors advise their diabetic patients to try and keep the blood sugar as near normal as possible and the urine mostly free from sugar. In some diabetic patients, this is not possible to achieve without the constant risk of hypoglycaemic reactions. These reactions are not only bad for the morale but are also detrimental to ultimate health. The real skill in the management of diabetes is to avoid too high blood sugars on the one hand and troublesome hypoglycaemic reactions on the other.

EMPLOYMENT

When we talk about good control or stabilization of diabetes, we mean the maintenance of a steady weight at a normal level, with urine largely free from sugar but without frequent hypoglycaemic reactions. The patient should be leading a normal life and enjoying a useful occupation.

There are very few employments that are denied to the diabetic. It is unwise for a young diabetic patient taking insulin to be involved in work which would endanger his own safety or the safety of others if he suffered loss of consciousness due to a hypoglycaemic reaction. In other words, it would be quite inappropriate for a patient taking insulin to be a steeplejack or to work on high scaffolding, nor should he be employed at a job in which he is in proximity to or in control of moving machinery. The dangers of driving a car are minimal for most insulin-dependent diabetics, but dangers do exist, and for any long-distance lorry driver the need to take insulin might constitute a real hazard. In practice, diabetics taking insulin have been employed in all sorts of occupations such as those mentioned, even including charge of a signal-box at a busy railway junction, and no untoward effects have occurred. Nevertheless, the risk is there and should be avoided. Shift work provides another problem. A nurse requiring insulin for diabetes may find her routine seriously upset if she has to go on to night duty, since the pattern of meals and insulin is considerably disturbed. Here again, although shift work is undesirable, many diabetic patients have managed very well with appropriate adjustment of meal and insulin schedule. It is easy enough to recommend a change of occupation, but this advice is not always easy to follow for a man who has been doing a job for many years, and is skilled at it. The upset of seeking new training and employment may do more harm than good.

In general, employers are no longer afraid to employ patients with diabetes since they realize that diabetic patients taking insulin are no more likely to be off work or unwell than their other employees. In fact, it can be shown that diabetics taking insulin lose less time off work because they are more conscientious about their reputation than non-diabetics as far as health is concerned.

HOLIDAYS

Holidays should provide no real difficulty. Once the principles of the diet are understood, it is usually fairly easy to enjoy the right type of meal even abroad with language difficulties. On the whole, in most countries, simple foods are always available and foreign fish contain just as much protein as do those from our own shores. A knowledge of the equivalent carbohydrate values of such foods as spaghetti and rice makes it easy to equate these with our more familiar bread and potatoes. It is best to avoid sweets and puddings but advantage can be taken of local fresh fruit, vegetables and cheeses.

Of course it is of first importance to take an adequate supply of appropriate insulin and a secure case for syringes and needles. Disposable syringes with needles attached are particularly helpful on holiday since they are lightweight and contained in sterile envelopes. Certainly, it is essential for the diabetic traveller not to be parted from his insulin and injection equipment, even if it means having two separate kits. This is particularly important when travelling by air when the main baggage is removed on checking in and has been known to go astray. An emergency kit should always be carried in the hand baggage.

Insulin is a very hardy hormone and withstands reasonable extremes of temperature without losing potency. It is best kept in a cool place and most hotels will keep some bottles not in use in the hotel refrigerator – but not in the freezer compartment. When touring in really hot countries, a useful tip is to carry the insulin bottles in cotton wool in a thermos flask, if possible cooled in the fridge overnight.

Many countries require travellers to be inoculated and there is no reason why this should disturb the diabetic. However, it is a good idea to get this over and done with a few weeks before going abroad since, occasionally, inoculation leads to a mild constitutional upset with a rise of temperature.

One of the difficulties that air travel offers to the diabetic is the disturbance of meal schedules, particularly when flying east to west or vice versa. For example, when flying to the United States the day is prolonged by some 6 hours and an extra meal is taken. This is best covered by an extra injection of insulin, preferably of a short acting insulin, before the last meal of the day. The amount of insulin given can be determined by a urine test. If the urine contains more than 2% sugar, a fifth (20%) of the normal day's insulin can be given additionally, and proportionately less if the sugar content is less than 2%. On the return trip, a main meal is lost and the total daily insulin dose should be reduced by a fifth. Hypoglycaemic reaction must be guarded against by taking extra sugar if in doubt.

When travelling abroad, the Medic-Alert bracelet or disc should be carried, as well as a card stating boldly that the bearer is diabetic and giving details of the insulin used (see page 99). This is a safeguard against the unlikely event of loss of consciousness due to hypoglycaemia.

The parents of a diabetic child or the spouse of a diabetic adult needing insulin may feel vulnerable when going on holiday lest a severe hypoglycaemic attack occur and sugar cannot be administered. In this case, it may be useful to take a glucagon kit (see page 99) as a precaution.

MEDICAL SUPERVISION

Every diabetic taking insulin should attend his doctor or a hospital clinic at regular intervals for supervision. Although some diabetics who have been taking insulin for several years may feel they can manage perfectly well without medical care, in practice adjustments in the regime have to be made from time to time and the visit to the clinic offers an opportunity for an assessment of any adjustments to be made. The urine tests will be supplemented by a blood sugar estimation and this is a valuable additional guide to good control. Regular weighing is of considerable importance. Undue increase in weight has to be guarded against, and it is surprising how insidiously this can occur unless weighings are regular. Increase in weight usually represents too high an intake of carbohydrate food and usually responds to adjustment of the diet and insulin in this respect. Undue loss of weight may be due to poor control of the diabetes with elevated blood sugars and may be an indication of some underlying infection. Pulmonary tuberculosis used to be very common in diabetes and must always be guarded against by a routine chest X-ray, even though it is seen less now than in the past.

The visit to the doctor or clinic offers the patient the opportunity of raising any questions concerning his diabetic routine or his general health. He achieves a rapport with his doctor and the records of his progress will show whether there has been any change in his general health that needs adjustment of the routine or additional treatment.

DRIVING A CAR

When applying for a driving licence, various questions have to be answered on eyesight and physical and mental capacity to drive a motor vehicle. Question 6 (d) includes the specific question: "Have you any defect or disability which could affect your fitness as a driver now or in the future?" and since diabetes comes within this definition, the answer must be 'yes'. Details are then required, and this means stating whether the diabetes is treated with insulin, tablets or diet alone. On returning the completed application form, a supplementary form may be received requesting the name and address of your doctor. So long as the doctor is prepared to confirm that the diabetes is well controlled and there are no complications which could impair safety as a driver, the licence to drive will be issued.

The real danger to diabetics in driving a car is the risk of a hypoglycaemic reaction while driving and loss of control. This could constitute a terrible risk not only to the driver but to others as well. Hence a diabetic who takes insulin should not drive a car or motorbike unless he has learned to recognize the symptoms of hypoglycaemia in good time to take proper action. He must understand when these reactions are liable to occur and never to drive when a mealtime is overdue. He must always carry sugar on his person and in the car. At the first sign of a reaction, he must draw into the side and take some sugar. The driving seat should be vacated and the ignition key removed to avoid the suggestion of being in charge of a car while in an unfit state. It is best to carry a disc or bracelet, such as that supplied by Medic-Alert, displaying the identity of the wearer and the fact that he has diabetes. Driving does not constitute a risk to diabetics on tablets nor to most well-controlled diabetics taking insulin. However, through no fault of their own, some diabetics on insulin are liable to frequent reactions, sometimes without warning. In their own interest as well as of others, they should not drive.

9

HYPOGLYCAEMIA AND DIABETIC COMA

HYPOGLYCAEMIA

Perhaps the one thought which most worries diabetic patients is the fear of hypoglycaemic reactions and the danger of losing consciousness. In fact, actual loss of consciousness is unusual in diabetics taking insulin and very exceptional indeed in patients taking tablets; but it is essential for every diabetic taking insulin to be aware of the early symptoms of hypoglycaemia and to take necessary action in good time.

Shortly after the discovery of insulin, Banting began to appreciate that if too much insulin was injected, the sugar in the blood became too low and unpleasant symptoms were liable to occur. The brain and the nervous system need a constant supply of glucose from the blood, and this can only be provided when the level of sugar in the blood is sufficient. Normally, the fasting level of sugar in the blood seldom falls below 80 mg/ml, though under certain circumstances it may fall lower than this even in good health. After vigorous exercises, such as a cross-country run or after rowing in a race, the sugar in the blood tends to fall because of the increased metabolism, but there are balancing factors which can elevate the blood sugar back to normal. Similarly, after prolonged starvation although the sugar in the blood tends to be on the low side, compensatory production of glucose from the liver stores soon offsets the deficit. Consequently, although in normal health the blood sugars may temporarily fall too low after violent exercise or prolonged starvation, this situation seldom gives rise to symptoms of hypoglycaemia.

There is no exact level at which a hypoglycaemic reaction will occur. In the main, most people can tolerate a blood sugar as low as 50 mg/100 ml without trouble but levels below this are very liable to give reactions. Coma is likely to ensue when the blood sugar level falls below 30 mg/100ml, but here again there is a good deal of personal variation. Some patients seem better able to tolerate low blood sugar levels without any symptoms, whereas others begin to get vague symptoms when the blood sugar level is hardly below normal. Unfortunately, the symptoms of hypoglycaemic reactions are not sufficiently precise to make the diagnosis an absolute one and nervous patients are more liable to be sensitive in this respect.

SYMPTOMS

The symptoms of hypoglycaemia in patients taking insulin vary to some extent according to the type of insulin injected and to personal idiosyncrasy.

Soluble insulin acts quickly and tends to lower the blood sugar more precipitously than the long-acting insulins. The earliest symptoms are those of weakness, trembling, sweating, visual blurring, tingling in the lips or mouth, a feeling of fear or hunger, and a general sense of something being wrong. Each patient will soon learn which particular symptoms herald an attack since there is no uniformity of reaction. In long acting insulins, the reduction of blood sugar may be much slower and the effects somewhat different. Slurring of speech and retardation of thought and action may be the first signs. Uncoordination of the limbs may occur with unsteadiness of gait. There may be confusion of thought and jumbling of words. Very commonly, changes in mood may occur with obstreperous behaviour and an unreasonable attitude. In this state the patient may be unaware of his situation and may become unco-operative in any attempts to treat it. Very often indeed the patient himself may not be the best guide as to what is going on and may well resist taking appropriate treatment on the grounds that there is nothing wrong. Particularly if he happens to have had a recent drink, making the breath smell of alcohol, this situation is easily mistaken for drunkenness and has even led to detention in a prison cell for the night with diasastrous results.

Particularly in children, hypoglycaemia may result in convulsive attacks which can be mistaken for epilepsy. To make matters more difficult, children may occasionally suffer from both diabetes and epilepsy. In this situation if the blood sugar falls too low it is liable to precipitate an epileptic attack.

If hypoglycaemia is not treated, recovery may be spontaneous with compensatory mechanisms raising the blood sugar to normal. However, often the effect of the injected insulin continues to dominate and the blood sugar falls still lower until the brain is unable to function adequately and a loss of consciousness ensues. Under these circumstances, the patient will be breathing quietly, the skin will be warm and moist, and the appearance that of someone in a deep sleep. Unless treatment is given this position can become serious since damage to the brain could result if it persists for many hours without treatment. Complete recovery can be expected in most cases, even when coma has persisted for as long as seven or eight hours.

Hypoglycaemic reactions in patients taking tablets are exceptional but occasionally occur when large doses are taken. For example, three tablets of 500 mg tolbutamide taken in a single dose in the morning has been found to give hypoglycaemic reactions of sweating, tremulousness and weakness. If the tablets are given all together before breakfast, these symptoms are liable to occur before lunch. However, if the tablets are spaced throughout the day, one before each meal, then reactions of this sort hardly ever happen. With the stronger tablets, such as chlorpropamide, hypoglycaemic effects are liable to occur in patients who are elderly or frail, particularly late at night. Cases of actual hypoglycaemic coma are very rare in patients taking tablets for diabetes, but may occur when other tablets have been taken which potentiate the hypoglycaemic effects of the sulphonylureas. For example, certain tablets taken for gout, blood pressure or depression may have this effect and it is as well for any patient taking the sulphonylureas to be aware of this risk. Phenformin and metformin do not cause the blood sugar to fall below normal and so offer no hazard in this respect.

CAUSES OF HYPOGLYCAEMIA

Hypoglycaemic attacks, sometimes known as 'reactions' or 'hypos', may occur for a variety of reasons.

1. MISTAKES IN INSULIN DOSAGE

Insulin is prepared commonly in two strengths, 40 and 80 units/ml. Clearly, if the 80 strength is used in error instead of the 40 strength, double the dose of insulin may be inadvertently taken. The syringe is another source of error. The standard BS1619 syringe has 20 marks to the millilitre but many other syringes are available with different markings, so that the wrong dose of insulin could be drawn up. Insulin itself may provide difficulties since, although standardized as to potency, in some individuals insulin prepared from pigs may be more effective than that prepared from cattle. This is because bovine insulin is more antigenic than porcine, and so may lead to the formation of antibodies which block its effect. Consequently, if one batch of insulin contains more porcine than bovine insulin, it may have a stronger action and could actually lead to hypoglycaemic reactions. On the whole, this effect is not a very important one in most patients, but cases have occurred where a change from a batch of insulin containing a higher proportion of porcine than bovine insulin has led to a substantial fall in blood sugar levels. We have only become aware of this difficulty in recent years and insulin is now available which has been extracted entirely from pigs.

2. CHANGE IN REQUIREMENTS

When young patients develop diabetes they are often underweight and the urine contains acetone as well as sugar. Large quantities of insulin are necessary to restore the metabolism to normal. If initial treatment is begun in hospital, the patient is at rest and taking very little exercise. Consequently, the dose of insulin needed in hospital is often considerably greater than ultimately becomes necessary when the patient leaves hospital, leads a more active existence and perhaps needs less food. Unless the dosage of insulin is reduced in accordance with these diminishing needs, hypoglycaemic reactions are very liable to occur. On the other hand, insulin requirements very often increase during an infection, after an accident or during pregnancy. Unless the insulin dosage is steadily reduced again when the situation has reverted to normal, the liability to hypoglycaemia will occur. It should be realized that insulin requirements are not fixed for all time and adjustments will have to be made according to circumstances.

3. FOOD HABITS

Undoubtedly, the commonest cause of reactions is irregularity in food habits. Since the insulin injected goes on exerting its effect in lowering the blood sugar even though no food is eaten, it is easily understood that a delay in taking food will lead to hypoglycaemia. A patient who normally has lunch at 1 p.m. and is delayed at the office may find himself having a hypoglycaemic reaction in the bus on his way home to lunch. In general, most diabetics taking insulin are well advised to have snack meals in addition to the three main meals of the day. A cup of coffee and a biscuit between breakfast and lunch, a light tea between lunch and supper, and a snack last thing at night are useful ways of maintaining a steady intake of carbohydrate fuel throughout the day.

4. EXERCISE

Most of us tend to undertake the same sort of activity from day to day and only occasionally participate in strenuous exercise. This is not to be deprecated since it is far better to take exercise sporadically than not at all. However, undue activity certainly burns up extra sugar and causes the insulin which has been injected to be absorbed more quickly. These effects may lead to hypoglycaemia unless particular care is taken to anticipate and prevent the blood sugar falling too low. In some patients hypoglycaemia seems to occur at weekends, even when there is no evidence that there has been an increase of physical activity during this time. This is sometimes difficult to explain but many diabetics have learned to take extra food at weekends for this reason.

5. SITE OF INJECTION

If insulin is always injected into the same area, the subcutaneous tissue becomes thickened and hard. The insulin injected there may be slowly absorbed but if the injection is just outside the particular area, absorption may be more rapid and complete. Variations of this sort can cause fluctuations in blood sugar levels.

6. UNKNOWN CAUSES

It must be understood that quite apart from the factors mentioned there are many other influences which affect blood sugar levels over which the patient has no control. For example, fluctuations in the blood sugar levels may be due to changes in menstrual pattern or other hormonal disturbances, and it is certainly true that emotion can play an important role. It is as well to stress this point since many diabetics suffering from reactions tend to blame themselves unnecessarily, failing to realize that even rigid adherence to the regime does not afford complete immunity from considerable fluctuations in blood sugar levels.

TREATMENT

The most important approach in the avoidance of hypoglycaemic reactions is for the patient to be aware of the causes, the symptoms and the treatment once symptoms appear. At the first sign of trouble, sugar or glucose must be taken forthwith. There is no particular harm in taking sugar unnecessarily from time to time, but there is every harm in delay when the blood sugar falls too low. Continued lowering of blood sugar levels may rob the patient of clear thinking and initiative, so that unless action is taken straight away, it may soon become too late. Every patient taking insulin must always have sugar available, usually in the form of wrapped glucose or wrapped lump sugar. Some should be kept in every jacket or handbag so that there is no need to transfer sugar from jacket to jacket when clothes are changed. Sugar must be kept easily to hand in the home and in the car.

It is important not only for patients to recognize the symptoms and treatment of hypoglycaemia but also for those living with them. This is particularly true for the wife or husband of a diabetic patient since unless action is taken in good time, obstructive behaviour or drowsiness may make it difficult to administer sugar. At the first sign of trouble, a cup of warm tea with two spoonsful of sugar should be given but sometimes considerable persuasion may be necessary before the patient will accept that this is necessary. If unconsciousness is beginning to ensue and the patient will not take sugar or a drink, syrup may be smeared on the inside of the mouth. This will lead to salivation and swallowing. If the patient is comatose, medical aid should be sought as soon as possible. It is dangerous to delay too long. When the patient arrives in hospital, the treatment of hypoglycaemic coma usually consists of the injection of sugar solutions into the vein. The effect is magical. As the injection is proceeding the patient starts to recover consciousness and soon begins to remember what led to the attack. Once immediate recovery has taken place, it is best to follow up with a meal since the short-lived benefit of the glucose injection will be offset by the continuing insulin effect, unless further carbohydrate is provided.

Clearly, the dangers of hypoglycaemic reactions offer a problem to the parents of children with diabetes when on holiday, perhaps out of reach of a doctor. Happily, there is now available in a form suitable for injection a hormone known as glucagon which has an effect entirely opposite to that of insulin and actually causes an elevation of the blood sugar level. Glucagon does not keep well in solution as does insulin, and so is prepared in powder form. This has to be dissolved in water and the solution then injected. The powder is contained in a sealed vial and 1 ml of sterile water is provided in another vial. The glass tops of both vials are easily broken, the sterile water is drawn into the syringe and this is now squirted into the vial containing the powder until it is fully dissolved. The resultant solution is drawn into the syringe and can be injected subcutaneously or into the muscle, as is insulin. This injection leads to an improvement in the blood sugar levels in about a quarter of an hour with return of consciousness, usually sufficient to enable the patient to be given a sweetened drink and a carbohydrate meal. It is wise to take glucagon on holiday in preparation for this possible emergency.

Every diabetic taking insulin must carry a card which makes clear that he or she has diabetes and advising the need for immediate transfer to hospital if found unconscious. There is also an organization known as Medic-Alert which provides an emblem in the form of a disc worn on a stainless steel chain bracelet. This contains the patient's number and the telephone number of the organization. The Medic-Alert Foundation maintains a central file which records information regarded by the patient's doctor as essential for adequate protection. This information can be obtained by making a reverse charge telephone call from anywhere in the world. The telephone is manned day and night and the information recorded at the central register is provided by the member in conjunction with his doctor, usually consisting of the amount and type of insulin which is injected each day and any other relevant information.

DIABETIC COMA

As has already been discussed, loss of consciousness can occur when the blood sugar falls too low but the term diabetic coma refers to exactly the opposite effect. In this case, the coma is due primarily to a considerable excess of sugar in the blood, though the accumulation of acetone which occurs at the same time may be equally important in some cases. These two factors in varying degrees lead to loss of consciousness since the functioning of the brain is impaired by the excess of sugar and acetone. The condition of diabetic coma is a very serious one and without vigorous and early treatment in hospital, death will inevitably ensue as it did so invariably in the days before insulin became available.

The onset of diabetic coma is gradual and is preceded by symptoms of uncontrolled diabetes. There is usually a loss of energy and weight with increasing thirst and polyuria. Vomiting may occur and the urine contains heavy amounts of sugar and acetone. Diabetic coma will only ensue when the diabetes has been getting out of control with steadily rising blood levels and production of ketones. Unlike hypoglycaemia, which usually happens very suddenly in somebody previously well, the onset of diabetic coma is the culmination of an increasing deterioration of the diabetes and general health.

Diabetic coma is most often precipitated by an infection so that there is often a history of some illness associated with the worsening of the diabetes. The infection is usually more than a minor one. A severe bout of tonsillitis, an attack of pneumonia, a bout of enteritis or an infection in the urinary tract (pyelitis) are common infections which may cause loss of control in the diabetic state. The condition is inevitably exacerbated if the patient goes off his food and erroneously assumes that as a result he does not need insulin. Nothing is more likely to induce coma than omission of the insulin in the face of illness. In fact, under these circumstances more and more ketones are produced and the blood sugar rises steadily despite the absence of food. The body actually breaks down its own stores of fat and protein as a source of fuel with the production of excessive sugar and ketones. Insulin is the only remedy for this serious metabolic disorder. Patients with diabetes are always urged to maintain or even to increase their insulin injections when they fall ill. Even if the normal full diet cannot be taken glucose drinks or light frequent feeds of carbohydrate food can and must be taken. The degree to which the insulin is increased will be dictated by the urinary tests and it is always wise to seek medical advice under these circumstances.

Although infection is the commonest precipitating cause of diabetic coma, ignorance and carelessness may also lead to this state. The proper care of diabetes needs a certain degree of intelligence and self-discipline and if these virtues are in short supply poor control of the diabetes is liable to occur with the dangers of infection and ultimate coma.

Occasionally the onset of coma is the first intimation of diabetes and this is particularly true of children. So often the parents have not noticed the increasing thirst and polyuria, and the onset of an infectious illness further masks the true nature of the condition. The symptoms may be ascribed to the infection, and coma may ensue before either parent or doctor becomes aware of the true nature of the under-lying condition. Diabetes is very unusual in small children and for this reason its presence is seldom suspected.

The earliest signs of diabetic coma are an increase in the symptoms of diabetes with thirst and polyuria often accompanied by vomiting and deepening of the breathing. The change in respiration is brought about by the increased production of ketones which are partly excreted in the breath. This gives the breath a characteristic odour, sometimes likened to new-mown hay or rotting apples.

The picture of a patient in diabetic coma is a very characteristic one. There is often a good deal of wasting of the musculature and the skin is dry and loose. The face is shrunk with a shrivelled, leathery tongue. The breathing is deep and sighing, and the breath smells of acetone. The extremities are cold and the doctor will observe that the pusle is rapid and thready with a low blood pressure. As soon as the patient is admitted to hospital, blood is drawn from the vein to esti-mate the amount of sugar present. There is no absolute level at which coma occurs, since the onset of coma is also dependent on the degree of acidity caused by the presence of ketones. Usually, however, the blood sugar level exceeds 600 mg/100 ml and may be considerably more.

Treatment is best carried out in hospital. In the first place, fluid must be given into the vein. This is necessary to replace the fluid loss occasioned by the excessive loss of urine over the preceding days. Since the patient is unconscious, he cannot be given fluid by mouth and consequently the venous route is chosen. Nowadays, specially prepared solutions of salt and alkalies are already prepared and sterilized and are allowed to drip slowly via a needle or fine tube inserted into the vein. The amount of fluid given can be estimated by various tests on the blood and urine, but a severe case may need several litres in the first few hours. The second essential treatment is insulin and this has to be administered both subcutaneously and into the vein. Soluble insulin is always used in these circumstances since its effect is the most immediate in reducing the level of sugar in the blood. Since the patient is so dehydrated and the circulation so poor, the insulin injected under the skin is poorly absorbed initially and for this reason insulin must also be given directly into the vein for a quicker effect. A third important aspect of treatment is the search for infection which may lie hidden in the middle ear, in the lungs or in the kidneys. Many physicians prefer to give antibiotics as a routine even though there is no overt evidence of infection to be found. During the whole of this procedure, specimens of blood are sent to the laboratory for investigations as to progress. Diabetic coma cannot satisfactorily be managed without the resources of a hospital laboratory, though this often entails long sessions of night work for the technicians concerned, as well as for the nurses and doctors. As a rule, with continuing fluids, insulin and antibiotics, the patient starts to recover consciousness after 6–12 hours, though the time will vary according to the depth of coma and the initial degree of elevation of the blood sugars and ketones.

With modern treatment, the outlook for recovery is very good providing no serious complications have occurred during the illness. The older the patient, the less confident the outlook, since the greater the danger of such complications as coronary thrombosis or kidney failure during the stage of coma. Once consciousness has returned, fluid and light food can be given by mouth and injections of insulin regulated by the amount of sugar and acetone in the urine.

10

SOME SPECIAL SITUATIONS: CHILDREN, PREGNANCY, THE ELDERLY, ASSOCIATED ILLNESSES

❦

DIABETES IN CHILDREN

Diabetes is uncommon in childhood and very unusual indeed in babies. It occurs equally in boys and girls and the commonest age of onset is about 12 years old.

CAUSE

Heredity appears to play a more important part in the onset of diabetes in children than it does in adults. The incidence of diabetes in the family of a child with diabetes is something like twenty times as great as occurs in the family of a child without diabetes. However, heredity is certainly not the only factor and many children who develop diabetes have no-one in their family with this complaint at all. It seems extraordinary that a child can suddenly develop diabetes without any family history and without any evidence of any antecedent cause. Infection of the pancreas is always a possible cause and occasionally it can be demonstrated that mumps has been responsible. The virus of mumps usually infects the parotid glands in the face, giving rise to the characteristic swelling over the jaws. Occasionally this stage is followed by severe abdominal pain, vomiting, and a further rise of temperature. These symptoms suggest an inflammation of the pancreatic gland similar to that which has occurred in the parotids and are sometimes followed by the onset of diabetes. This is a rare occurrence but much research has gone into the possibility of other types of virus infection which could cause diabetes in children, so far without much success. Of course, infection may bring to light an underlying diabetes and exacerbate the symptoms. For example, a child may have mild diabetes with minimal symptoms, but the onset of tonsillitis may precipitate the illness into a more severe state.

The discovery of diabetes in a child is usually a severe blow to the parents and they are naturally anxious as to the child's future. It can be said at the outset that children with diabetes who are properly treated develop in a normal way. Their height and growth is strictly comparable with non-diabetic children, and their mental development is in all ways similar. In girls who develop diabetes before puberty, the onset of the period is sometimes delayed for a year or two, but this is not always the case and has no serious significance.

The onset of diabetes in children is usually more abrupt than in adults. Symptoms of thirst and polyuria are more insistent, and bedwetting is a common feature. The child may seem tired and lustreless and although he may eat very well, he may actually lose weight. Unless the condition is diagnosed at this stage, drowsiness with a tendency to fall asleep may be noticed. Often this is followed by nausea or vomiting and these symptoms may lead to actual coma with deep sighing breathing and a smell of acetone in the breath. Because diabetes is so unusual in children, the diagnosis is often delayed because the parents are unaware of this possibility. Testing of the urine by the doctor will soon reveal the true situation since both sugar and acetone will be present. The diagnosis can be confirmed by a glucose tolerance test but this is seldom necessary in children since the diagnosis is usually obvious from the general picture, the finding of sugar in the urine and a single blood test which usually reveals a greatly elevated level of sugar.

The aims of treatment of diabetes in children is in two main directions. Firstly, the child must be relieved of symptoms, and be able to lead a full and happy life at home and at school. The second aim of treatment is to safeguard the future and to ruduce the risks of ill health in later life. In the present state of our knowledge this is best achieved by keeping the blood sugar levels as near normal as possible but without the disadvantages of frequent hypoglycaemic reactions. These two ambitions are in some ways contradictory since the blood sugar levels tend to fluctuate during the day. Attempts to keep the urine free from sugar all the time may well lead to frequent hypoglycaemic reactions, a very undesirable state of affairs.

The diet for children must be related both to the home circumstances and to the school. It is of prime importance for the parent and for the child to understand the features of the diet and the relative importance of carbohydrates proteins and fats. There is no doubt that the most fruitful time for instruction is as soon as possible after diagnosis has been made. The child should learn which are the carbohydrate foods and should have a clear idea of how much he is allowed at each meal. As usual, this is best done by finding out what his normal eating habits have been and adjusting the diet to alter these habits as little as possible. School meals provide some difficulty but if the child knows how much bread or potato he is allowed, he can usually manage reasonably well. It may be necessary to provide him with biscuits and cheese or with fruit as an alternative to the pudding. The question of sweets and chocolates is a difficult one. It should be explained that sweets and chocolates cause the sugar in the blood to accumulate too quickly and this is ultimately harmful to good health. In the end it is the child's own good sense that matters and attempts at policing the child too rigidly will inevitably lead to failure. Diabetic chocolates are available. They have a calorie value but are helpful as an alternative to ordinary chocolates since they do not contain any sugar. There is no drastic damage done if the child has occasional sweets or chocolates, but if the attitude is too lax in this respect, control of the diabetes is likely to be impaired with bad results in the years ahead. Apart from anything else, it is generally accepted that excessive eating of sweets and chocolates is unhealthy and in particular disposes to caries of the teeth. Ice cream and other extras are easily introduced into the diet since their calorie value is known and can replace other foods.

The important rules of diet are those of regularity both in amount and in timing. The three main meals of the day should be taken at about the same time and snacks should be provided between breakfast and lunch, between lunch and supper, and last thing at night. School-teachers should be aware that a diabetic child must not be kept in late if this interferes with his mealtimes.

Almost all children who develop diabetes need insulin. As a rule, when diabetes is first diagnosed, large amounts are necessary to control the metabolic disorder. The dose of insulin then tends to diminish until in fact many children go through a phase when they need very little or no insulin at all. At this stage, treatment by tablets is sometimes possible but unfortunately the success is usually only short-lived. After a variable time, the diabetes will require insulin injections again. In the face of these facts, most physicians prefer to keep children on small doses of insulin even during a phase when very little is needed. This avoids the disappointment that otherwise ensues if insulin has been discontinued and then has to be reintroduced.

The type of insulin to be used and the frequency of injection are matters which must be decided for each individual case. In the main, there is a consensus of opinion that insulin given twice a day offers better health in the long term than a single injection. Many children are well controlled by an injection of soluble insulin twenty minutes before breakfast and another injection twenty minutes before supper. If on this regime the urine shows sugar in the afternoon or in the early morning, it may be useful to add a long acting insulin to the morning or evening soluble insulin. Thus, control may be achieved by a mixture of 20 units soluble insulin with 10 units isophane insulin in the morning, and another injection of 16 units soluble insulin before the evening meal. There is no golden rule in this respect and many regimes using different kinds of insulin can all be successful.

Tablet treatment seldom controls diabetes in children except as a temporary phase, shortly after diagnosis. Nevertheless, some children have been managed on tablet treatment without resource to insulin at all, but it is not yet sure whether they will develop as normally as children taking insulin.

The urine should be tested regularly and when possible three times a day. A chart should be kept of the amount of sugar present since this is a very useful guide as to progress when it is shown to the doctor. On the whole, frequent adjustments of insulin are undesirable but if heavy amounts of sugar persist in the urine for several days it may be wise for the parent to temporarily increase the amount of insulin. Similarly, urine that is consistently free from sugar must alert the parents to the dangers of reactions and it may be necessary to reduce the insulin to avoid this situation.

Children with diabetes must not in any sense be regarded as ill or as invalids. They must be encouraged to take part in all school activities including games and physical exercise. It may be necessary to augment the diet with glucose sweets if exercise of unusual activity is to be undertaken. Once instruction has been given the child himself usually learns how to manage in this respect.

There is no particular age at which a child should learn to inject himself with insulin but in general most children at the age of 8 can manage quite successfully. Certainly, they can be instructed in the manoeuvres of drawing up the insulin at an early age, but there may be a natural reluctance to insert the needle under the skin. In fact, there are various types of apparatus available which may help the child to overcome his hesitation in this respect. The insulin gun is an apparatus which holds the syringe and needle and can be placed against the skin. When the trigger is pulled the needle is pushed under the skin and the injection can then be given. Mostly, although this apparatus may be helpful in the early stages, the child soon learns to inject himself without mechanical aids. Parents have a responsibility to instruct the diabetic child to inject himself since if they are over-indulgent in this respect the child may become too dependent on his parents with loss of independence and self-reliance.

Hypoglycaemic reactions are troublesome and destructive of morale. A diabetic child at school who loses consciousness due to an insulin reaction causes a great deal of excitement and unwanted attention. It is disturbing to the school-teacher who feels an added responsibility. Fortunately, with reasonable care, these reactions can be avoided and do not cause trouble in the large majority of children with diabetes. The urine tests form a good guide and the child must be carefully instructed as to the early symptoms of hypoglycaemia and as to what to do as soon as he gets the early sensations. He must always have wrapped sugar on his person and in his desk at school. It is much better for a child to take sugar unnecessarily than to run the risk of a hypoglycaemic reaction. The parents must be on the lookout for early symptoms and these are particularly liable to occur before mealtime and especially if the child has undertaken unusual activity. When on holiday it is wise to take ampoules of glucagon so that an injection can be given if there is a severe reaction and the child is unable to swallow a sweetened drink or to take sugar. An injection of glucagon will usually lead to a return to consciousness within twenty minutes and a sweetened drink with some bread and butter can then be given. Frequent hypoglycaemic reactions usually necessitates an adjustment of the insulin dose and of eating habits.

When a diabetic child falls ill with an infection such as measles or tonsillitis, the parents must be aware of the fundamental importance of injecting insulin even though the child is unable to eat his usual food. Ketones will quickly form in the blood if insulin is not given and indeed, this is a frequent cause of diabetic coma. Sweetened drinks can usually be administered without trouble and provide an adequate substitute for food under these circumstances. No attempt should be made to stick rigidly to the usual diet. Any food that the child will tolerate should be given when he is ill with an infectious fever or a raised temperature from any cause. Fluids must be given in plenty and if the urine shows excess sugar the insulin dose may have to be increased on medical advice.

There is no doubt that diabetes imposes a psychological strain both on the child and the parents. From the child's viewpoint, the denial of many foods and sweets of which he may be particularly fond and which he sees other children eating offers a sense of deprivation if he adheres to the rules and a feeling of guilt if he does not. The morning ritual of insulin injection and the testing of urine during the day can become detestable and many diabetic children either go through a stage of active rebellion in which they refuse to inject themselves or through a stage of passive resistance with a sullen and resentful attitude. The child may subconsciously blame his parents for the ailment and for the restrictions that it entails.

From the parents' viewpoint, there is often a sense of guilt and a feeling that in some unspecified way the onset of diabetes may have occurred through some fault or omission of their own. However illogical this may be, this feeling is often strengthened by the need to impose unwelcome restrictions on the child they love. Torn between the natural desire to be indulgent and loving on one hand and the fear of harming the child's future through a failure to adhere to the regime on the other, the parents may well develop a feeling of insecurity and tension. Despite all these possibilities, happily in most cases parents and child soon become adjusted to the needs and realities of the situation so that in practice diabetic children mostly lead a normal and active life at home and at school.

Nevertheless, diabetes imposes a strain both on the psychological stability and adaptability of the family and where these virtues are in short supply, the situation may become intolerable. A maladjusted child with unintelligent parents simply cannot manage the diabetic routine without frequent admissions to the hospital either with hypoglycaemic reactions or with diabetic coma. Although fortunately this situation is not a common one, there are sufficient numbers of diabetic children in this category to warrant the setting up of special homes for the residential care of these children where they can be trained in their routine and encouraged by the proximity of others needing the same discipline.

In a much happier setting, the British Diabetic Association has also organized holiday camps and cruises for healthy and well-adjusted diabetic children. These have proved a great success in that the youngsters soon learn that they are not isolated by their diabetes but that many other children have the same disability and manage with success. Nothing is more likely to give a child confidence than to see other children of the same age injecting themselves, testing their own urine, and observing a sensible diet. Life at a diabetic camp or on a holiday cruise is no different from that enjoyed by other children on holiday. The diabetic children play the same games and enjoy the sea and the sun as uninhibited as any other children.

The onset of puberty may be a particularly trying time for the diabetic child and it is at this stage that rebellion most commonly occurs. Parents will know from experience with other children of the emotional upsets that are liable to occur at this stage of life in any youngster and there is no doubt that the presence of diabetes accentuates the emotional difficulties of this stage in growing up. An attitude compounded of firmness and explanation is the best to adopt. It must be stressed that without insulin no activity could be undertaken at all and that a life of invalidism would be the only alternative. Explanation must be made of the need to preserve good health for the future and although most young people are very averse to looking ahead (they would not smoke cigarettes if they did!) yet reference to the need to keep healthy in order to be married and support a family will often have a steadying effect.

DIABETES IN PREGNANCY

It has been found that women who are destined to develop diabetes in later life often have unusually large babies long before diabetes actually develops. These babies may weigh more than 10 lb and are some-times stillborn. Of course, big babies may be born to women who never develop diabetes but it happens sufficiently frequently to women who later become diabetic to make it quite clear that the ten-dency to diabetes has some effect on the child in the womb long before the sugar in the blood of the mother is noticeably raised. It looks as though there is much more to diabetes than an excess of sugar in the blood and just what the abnormality is has so far eluded discovery. It may be some hormonal dysfunction which itself later disposed to the onset of diabetes, or it may be part and parcel of a general disorder which ultimately causes the sugar to accumulate in the blood by re-stricting the output of insulin. Since women destined to develop dia-betes tend to have large babies, it is not surprising that women who have actually developed diabetes should show a tendency to produce large babies and an increased rate of stillborn babies. Although a raised blood sugar is clearly not the only cause, there is no doubt that these events are related to a large extent to the degree of elevation of sugar in the blood. Many studies have demonstrated that the better the diabetes is controlled throughout the pregnancy, the better the chances of a live and healthy baby. In fact, the incidence of stillborn babies in diabetic mothers who are well controlled is now not very much greater than in women without diabetes. In short, an otherwise healthy diabetic mother has every chance of having a normal baby and she need not face the pregnancy with undue apprehension, pro-viding she is prepared to adhere strictly to her diabetic regime.

Many mothers with diabetes worry lest the baby be born in some way deformed or especially liable to develop diabetes. In fact, such fears are groundless since there is no real evidence that congenital deformities are commoner in babies born of diabetic mothers. The incidence of diabetes itself in the offspring of mothers with diabetes is hardly higher than average, providing the father is a non-diabetic. Surprisingly, even if both parents have diabetes, the incidence of dia-betes in their children is only about 5%, so that this is not a very great risk.

The dangers to the health of the diabetic mother in having a baby are really very slight, providing she is under good supervision throughout the pregnancy from the aspect both of the diabetes and of her pregnancy. From the viewpoint of the diabetes, insulin requirements may need adjustment to attain more accurate control. Frequent and regular testing of the urine must be undertaken and a weekly visit to the clinic is advisable for blood sugar estimation. As soon as there is evidence that the sugar in the blood and urine is increasing, the dose of insulin must be adjusted accordingly. It is usually preferable to take insulin more than once a day during the pregnancy since an injection both morning and evening offers better control of the blood sugars. Even though the insulin requirements may increase considerably during the pregnancy, the dose may have to be lowered again once the baby is born, usually falling to the previous level. Providing the mother was in good health before the pregnancy, there is no evidence that the diabetes is made worse by pregnancy or that the expectation of good health is reduced by undergoing a pregnancy. Of course, a diabetic mother has the routine of her diabetic care to consider as well as that of looking after her baby. For this reason alone, it is usually considered inadvisable for a diabetic mother to have more than two children, though this is not an absolute rule.

The management of diabetes throughout the pregnancy depends on greater regularity in the diet, on frequent testing of the urine, and on insulin injections usually twice a day. As far as the diet is concerned, it is important for the expectant diabetic mother not to put on undue weight and to have an adequate intake of protein. In practice, this may mean some reduction of the carbohydrate intake and an increased amount of protein food in the form of milk, cheese, eggs, fish, poultry or meat. Regular weighing must be undertaken through the pregnancy and the weight compared with that which should be expected in a normal pregnancy. Any hint of undue weight may need reduction of the diet and possibly lowering of the insulin dose. As far as insulin is concerned, patients who have been managing well on a single injection a day of a long acting insulin may continue to do so, providing the evening specimens of urine are sugar free. If they are not, it is best to give an additional injection of insulin before the evening meal.

Diabetes is sometimes diagnosed when pregnancy has already begun. The presence of sugar in the urine during pregnancy is quite common and does not always represent diabetes. Sometimes in pregnancy, sugar appears very easily in the urine even though the sugar in the blood is normal. This so called low renal threshold is an innocent condition and does not require special treatment. Nevertheless, the finding of sugar in the water during pregnancy will usually call for a glucose tolerance test with blood sugar estimations to determine whether or not actual diabetes is present. Once it has been established that diabetes is present then the first step to be undertaken is dietary advice with a reduction of carbohydrate and general calorie intake. Sometimes, a diet which is adequate in protein but with a restricted carbohydrate intake is quite sufficient to restore the blood sugars to normal and in this case nothing more need be done apart from regular supervision.

If dietary restriction alone is not adequate to restore normoglycaemia (normal blood sugar), then the question arises as to whether tablets or insulin should be used. There is no evidence that the sulphonylureas are in any way harmful to the baby and many physicians use them successfully for control of the diabetes throughout pregnancy. In some cases, it has been shown that the blood sugar of the newborn baby falls too low just before delivery when the mother has been taking tablets, so that it is customary to omit the tablets just before delivery is due. This apart, sulphonylurea tablets can be used quite successfully during pregnancy, always providing that the blood sugars are maintained at a normal level. It certainly is quite mistaken to continue to rely on tablets unless normoglycaemia is being maintained. Many physicians prefer to use insulin rather than tablets if the blood sugars are not controlled on simple dietary restrictions, perhaps feeling that this is a safer and longer-established treatment than tablets.

It is not uncommon for a diabetic patient controlled on tablets to become pregnant, and here again the important question is whether or not the blood sugars are adequately controlled. If the tablets are indeed successful in maintaining normoglycaemia, then there seems no need to change over to insulin. Only if the blood sugars start to rise and the urine begins to show sugar should insulin be substituted.

The major disadvantage that diabetes imposes on the unborn baby is that of steadily increasing size during the last weeks of pregnancy, and it is for this reason that the mother must be under regular care by the obstetrician. He is in the best position to assess whether or not the foetus is becoming dangerously large during the later months of pregnancy, since experience has shown that increasing size of the unborn baby may lead to a stillborn baby. For this reason, it is a common practice in diabetic pregnancies deliberately to induce labour at about 36 to 38 weeks, several weeks before the baby would normally be born. The situation poses a real dilemma. If the pregnancy is allowed to continue to full term, there is a risk of a large, stillborn baby. If the baby is delivered too early, it may be too premature to survive. For this reason, considerable skill is necessary in deciding the best time to deliver the baby. The delivery itself may be effected either by inducing labour by a manoeuvre known as rupturing the membranes, or by a caesarean section in which the baby is removed from the uterus by an abdominal incision. Both methods can be equally successful but of course in either case if this is earlier than normal, the baby will be somewhat premature and may need special care by the paediatrician. The baby will probably be unable to feed at the breast and indeed the diabetic mother will probably not be able to provide an adequate supply of breast milk at this stage. This means that the infant will require tube feeding and may in addition need oxygen if its breathing is in any way impaired. This situation is best handled in a premature baby unit. Although this may sound extremely hazardous, in fact the results are very good and a diabetic mother who keeps to the rules can expect a healthy baby with reasonable confidence.

DIABETES IN THE ELDERLY

Diabetes can occur at any age and although the commonest onset is at about 40 or 50, it can certainly develop in the elderly. As a rule, diabetes in the elderly is quite mild and indeed it is very common for there to be some impairment of carbohydrate metabolism with growing age. The symptoms are similar to those occurring in younger people though in elderly women the irritation of pruritus vulvae is particularly common as a presenting symptom. As with younger patients, diabetes is commoner in those who are overweight and in these obese elderly patients a simple restriction of diet is all that is necessary to restore the blood sugar to normal. The basic requirements of treatment in the elderly are different from those in younger patients. In the elderly, fears of complications in the years ahead are hardly relevant and the stress is more on being able to lead an active and trouble-free life from day to day. Consequently, although there is not the same insistence on maintaining normoglycaemia, it is every bit as important to avoid troublesome symptoms and the dangers of infection that derive from an elevated sugar level in the blood.

Many elderly diabetics who are not well controlled on a simple dietary restriction will require tablets. There is little point in organizing a detailed weighed diet in older people since it is unlikely they will either have the will or the capacity to adhere to it. The sort of food they eat in the ordinary way should form the basis of their diet, with restriction on sugar, jam, and other foods rich in carbohydrate. Protein food should be encouraged to the limits of appetite and milk is particularly valuable in this respect. The choice of tablet will depend on the degree of obesity. In patients who are not overweight, the sulphonylureas are the best choice and probably tolbutamide is the safest tablet in old patients since its hypoglycaemic action is not so prolonged and not so severe as some of the longer acting tablets. Chlorpropamide tends to be too effective in elderly patients and may give rise to a low blood sugar during the night time, especially if the appetite has been poor and very little eaten for the evening meal. Tolbutamide is well tolerated and can be taken at breakfast or at supper.

In elderly patients who are obese, the biguanides are preferable to the sulphonylureas, since they help to keep down the weight as well as getting rid of the sugar. Unfortunately, they are not always acceptable since they make some patients feel rather ill with looseness of the bowel. Metformin can be given as a tablet after breakfast and after lunch. If it is well tolerated, it is extremely useful, particularly as it never causes the blood sugars to fall too low.

Urine testing in patients on tablets should be carried out by the Clinistix test and once a week is enough if the urine shows no sugar. If sugar is present, testing must be more frequent and may have to be done once or twice a day in order to provide a proper assessment for the doctor. If glycosuria is frequently present, blood sugar tests will need to be done from time to time to estimate whether or not the blood sugar is seriously elevated. Providing no symptoms are present, and providing the weight is at a reasonable level, the presence of sugar in the urine is not a cause for alarm in itself. Indeed, it might even be preferable for a slight amount of sugar to be present in the urine from time to time, particularly if the blood sugar levels are not considerably elevated, because there is then no danger of hypoglycaemia. Tablet therapy is particularly suitable for old people provided that they are under medical supervision. It is easy enough for an elderly man who lives on his own to take a tablet or two each day, and then to assume that this is all that is necessary. But unless supervision of the urine, weight, and blood is undertaken, his diabetic condition may deteriorate without his being aware of it. Consequently, although tablet treatment is convenient, it carries with it the onus of adequate supervision.

Insulin injections are not needed as commonly in elderly people as in younger ones, but certainly there are many older patients in whom tablet treatment is inadequate. These patients must have insulin and would soon lapse into ketosis and coma if it were not given. Insulin injections are usually very well managed by elderly patients, particularly if the diabetes came on when they were younger and so they had learned what to do when at a more adaptable age. It is more difficult for someone aged 70 to learn the routine of insulin injection, particularly if the eyesight is poor and the general health somewhat infirm. Under these circumstances, usually some other member of the family can perform the daily routine of insulin injection but if not, the district nurse is usually prepared to co-operate in this way. Indeed, one of the advantages of insulin as opposed to tablets for elderly patients living on their own is that a daily visit by the district nurse is extremely helpful, not only for the injection but for general supervisory purposes. Elderly diabetics living alone will usually need to attend a diabetic clinic if one is available and it may be possible to arrange for a social worker to call from time to time to make sure that all is going well.

The diet for the elderly patients on insulin must be given at regular intervals, with fairly regular amounts at each meal. This is usually easy to arrange when somebody else is present in the house who can supervise these matters but the situation is so difficult for some elderly infirm diabetic patients living on their own that sometimes residential care becomes obligatory. The diet need not be too formal, though clearly it is an advantage if the amount of carbohydrate eaten at each meal is fairly standardized. Unfortunately, the cost of a diabetic diet is something like 20% more than that usually eaten, largely because it contains more protein, and this can pose a burden on the elderly pensioner. Under the National Health Service, pensioners are relieved of all financial costs of tablets, syringes, insulin, spirit, cotton-wool and dressings.

Elderly diabetics have two disabilities particular to their age. Firstly, they are liable to poor vision, and secondly, they are prone to develop trouble with their feet.

Diabetes disposes to cataracts in the eyes and although cataracts are common in elderly non-diabetics experience seems to suggest that diabetes contributes to the development of this disorder. The visual deterioration that may occur with cataract formation makes it difficult for elderly patients to test the urine accurately for sugar or to draw up and inject insulin. Fortunately, the standard syringe (BS1619) has very clear markings especially designed for easy reading for patients with poor eyesight. The lens lies in the front part of the eye and concentrates light on to the retina. If the lens becomes opaque, light cannot get through and vision becomes correspondingly impaired. Cataract extraction is not difficult to perform these days and in most cases restores useful vision previously lost. Diabetes offers no real bar to operation, though special care is needed to maintain the blood sugar at a normal level after the operation has been performed. A raised blood sugar disposes to infection, which could be dangerous after operation when the eye is healing. Certainly any elderly diabetic whose vision is failing should seek advice as to the feasibility of operation and the opportunity of restored good eyesight.

Elderly diabetics are particularly prone to poor circulation in the feet. This is due to hardening of the arteries. In addition, changes in the nerves leads to impairment of sensation so that in many cases the feet are somewhat numb and insensitive to pain. As a result, minor injuries to the feet may pass unnoticed, and as the circulation is poor, serious damage may be done without the patient being in the least aware of it. Ulcers may occur on the toes and if infection sets in, which is particularly liable to occur if the diabetes is poorly controlled, local gangrene may follow. This means that the damage to the toe may become irreparable and surgical removal of the damaged area must be undertaken. To make matters worse, where vision is impaired the elderly diabetic may be unable to see clearly what is happening to the foot. This divorce of the diabetic from his feet means that special precautions must be adopted to avoid these disasters. Elderly diabetics must be encouraged to keep their feet as clean as they keep their face.

The skin must be carefully dried between the toes after washing. The shoes must be inspected before putting them on by placing a hand inside to make sure there are no rough places or protruding nails. The shoes should be comfortable and not tight fitting, with no places where rubbing takes place. Hot baths are best avoided since the numbness of the feet may not be able to perceive just how hot the water is. Similarly, on a cold day it is most undesirable for a diabetic to place the feet near a hot fire. Much better to allow them to warm gradually in a warm room. Elderly diabetics with poor eyesight should not cut their own toenails since the scissors may do damage when the feet are insensitive. If it is possible, a visit to the chiropodist from time to time is a very helpful procedure, particularly if corns need attention.

DIABETES IN ASSOCIATED ILLNESSES

On the whole, when the diabetes is well controlled, there is no particular reason why a diabetic patient should be more prone to infectious illnesses than anyone else. Indeed, surveys undertaken at diabetic clinics show that diabetic patients lose less time from work for mild infections than do others of the same age without diabetes. Perhaps this is because the diabetic patient looks after himself better and is more anxious to keep going unless really obliged to stay off work.

When infection occurs, such as a sore throat, a feverish cold, or a bowel infection, the diabetic patient is as well advised to rest in bed as anyone else. Antibiotic treatment may be thought necessary by the doctor and usually brings the infection under rapid control. One factor needs emphasis. If the normal diet cannot be eaten because of sickness or nausea, it is of paramount importance to maintain or increase the insulin dosage throughout the illness. Nothing is more liable to induce ketosis and coma than the omission of insulin in a patient with a temperature who is unable to take food and even more so if there is any vomiting. If food itself cannot be taken, the easiest substitute is to take drinks with sugar or glucose which is easy to tolerate. Some of the proprietary drinks containing glucose or dextrose are usually palatable even to someone who is feeling sick and has been vomiting.

If the diabetic patient is afflicted with a more chronic ailment such as coronary thrombosis, it is very usual for the insulin requirements to be increased in patients aleady on insulin, or for insulin treatment to become necessary in patients previously controlled on tablet treatment.

It is very important to try and keep the blood sugars as near normal as possible in patients going through an illness lasting several weeks. There is good evidence that recovery is delayed if the blood sugars are too elevated. This is equally true in patients who have undergone a surgical operation.

The care of the diabetic patient needing operation usually entails discussion between the physician, the anaesthetist and the surgeon. Where possible, the normal diet is adhered to for the days before the operation but usually nothing should be taken by mouth on the day of the operation itself. Instead, it is customary to provide fluid and dextrose directly into the bloodstream. A needle is inserted into the vein, not a difficult or a painful procedure, and suitable sterilized fluid is dripped in gradually from a bottle or plastic container. If the patient is on insulin, usually two-thirds of the normal dose is given before operation and blood sugar estimations are performed during and after the operation, in order to assess whether more insulin or more dextrose is needed. If the sugar in the blood is too low, more dextrose is given: if too high, more insulin is administered. On the day after the operation, where possible a light diet is arranged and no particular attempt is made to restrict the amount of carbohydrate, this being mostly a matter of what the patient is able to take. Insulin is usually given in divided doses during the day according to the urine and blood tests. As a rule, diabetic patients offer no difficulties when an operation is necessary, but supervision with laboratory backing is always necessary in insulin-dependent patients. Diabetics controlled by tablets or diet offer very little difficulty and it is usually quite safe to leave off tablets on the day of the operation so long as the urine tests are normal.

11

COMPLICATIONS OF DIABETES

EXPECTATION OF LIFE

Before the advent of antibiotics, the expectation of life of those who developed diabetes was considerably reduced compared with non-diabetics. Particularly when poorly controlled, diabetes reduces the resistance to infection and in the days before antibiotics were available, every illness offered a serious hazard to the diabetic. In no field was this more true than in tuberculosis, very much more common then than now. Every physician dreaded the onset of pulmonary tuberculosis in his diabetic patient because the prolonged infection in the lungs made the diabetes more difficult to control and the raised blood sugar had a bad effect on the tuberculosis infection. Diabetes and tuberculosis made a sinister combination. For a similar reason, particularly in elderly patients, infection of the lower limbs was very likely to lead to gangrene. Gangrene is a word used to denote loss of viability and occurs in a toe or foot when it is deprived of its blood supply by thickening or blockage of the artery: infection quickly sets in and gangrene results. Surgical operations were a more serious hazard in diabetics, partly because the anaesthesia was less safe and partly because infection could not be overcome. For example, an appendicitis would be a much more formidable and serious catastrophe in a diabetic in the days before antibiotics and the post-operative phase particularly hazardous if peritonitis was present. Diabetic coma was very much more common before the war than it is now because biochemical estimations were much less informative, methods of treatment were not so precise, and the advent of infection could not be effectively countered.

Childbearing in the diabetic mother carried a much higher mortality rate than now, again partly because of a poorer understanding of the factors involved and partly because of the inability to overcome the postpuerperal infections which used to be so common after childbirth in diabetic mothers.

The outlook in all these conditions today has vastly improved. Pulmonary tuberculosis, no longer described as consumption, is now fully treatable. Thanks to the advent of streptomycin and other similar drugs, tuberculosis has largely been eradicated and is curable when it occurs. The onset of tuberculosis in a diabetic patient no longer offers the same risks to the expectation of life, since both conditions can be kept under good control from their inception and providing treatment is thorough and prolonged, cure of the infection can be expected. Minor infections can be effectively treated from an early stage and since the discovery of the sulphonamides and penicillin, very few infections are allowed to spread. This is particularly important in elderly people with minor infection occurring in the feet so that gangrene can often be averted with proper supervision and early treatment.

Diabetic coma today is a comparative rarity and is usually found in three situations. Firstly, it sometimes happens that the diagnosis of diabetes has been unsuspected and the patient has lapsed into coma before the real state of affairs has been realized. Secondly, a very severe infection may lead to coma in a diabetic patient, either because the infection has not responded well to antibiotics or because the patient has not sought medical help before it was too late. Thirdly, it must be confessed that the care of diabetes demands a certain self-discipline and intelligence and without these virtues, poor control of the diabetes may ultimately lead to the onset of coma. With proper care, however, none of these factors occur very commonly and for this reason it is unusual for diabetic coma to be a cause of death today except in the very elderly or in those suffering from some other severe and untreatable ailment.

Now that these major hazards have been removed, the expectation of life of the man or woman who develops diabetes is scarcely less than that of the normal population, a fact supported by the willingness of many life insurance companies to accept diabetics at a near normal premium. The diabetic who looks after himself intelligently can expect to lead a full and healthy life.

CORONARY THROMBOSIS

The biggest cause of death in diabetics is that of coronary thrombosis. This ailment is becoming more common throughout the Western world and much research has gone into elucidating the various factors leading to this condition.

The heart is a muscular pump which contracts about seventy times a minute and is capable of doing so for over eighty years. Like all muscle, it must have a blood supply to carry oxygen and nutriment to it. The blood supply of the heart is carried by two small blood vessels arising from the aorta and known as the coronary arteries. These coronary arteries ramify throughout the muscle of the heart like the branches of a tree. Every muscle fibre of the heart must receive blood from twigs of the coronary branches. The coronary arteries themselves have a smooth inner lining, the endothelium, and it is this lining that gradually becomes thicker as we grow older. This process is known as arteriosclerosis and is largely due to deposition in the endothelium of substances containing cholesterol, itself partly derived from fats. When the endothelium of the coronary arteries becomes very thick it seriously impedes the flow of blood with the result that the musculature of the heart begins to suffer from an inadequate blood supply. From the patient's viewpoint, he may find that he is getting pain in the chest when he hurries, a symptom known as angina, and this is evidence that the heart is unable to fulfil its obligations when under stress because of the paucity of the blood supply.

These narrowed coronary arteries may in fact become blocked, either because some of the thickened endothelium becomes detached and so obliterates the lumen of the artery or because the blood flow through the narrowed artery is so sluggish that it forms a clot. In either case, obstruction of the artery means that part of the heart muscle is deprived of its vital oxygen supply. This area of the muscle may die, a process known as infarction, and depending on the amount of muscle involved, the patient will suffer accordingly. If a main branch of the coronary artery is blocked, the heart will fail completely and death will ensue. If a smaller branch is involved, the effect will not be serious at all and indeed may not be noticed. The usual symptoms of coronary thrombosis are those of a heavy pressing pain across the chest, sometimes going into the neck or down the left arm. Unlike angina, the pain may persist for several hours and usually comes on when the patient is at rest. Providing the infarct is not a large one, complete healing of the damaged area of the heart usually takes place, and the patient is able to resume normal activity.

Diabetes is a common predisposing cause of coronary thrombosis but by no means the only one. It has been convincingly demonstrated that the incidence of coronary thrombosis is partially related to the amount of sugar eaten. Refined sugar such as is eaten in the civilized world today is a highly unnatural food. It is absorbed too rapidly for the body's natural metabolism. Excess is converted to fat and perhaps this is the reason why excessive intake of sugar predisposes to

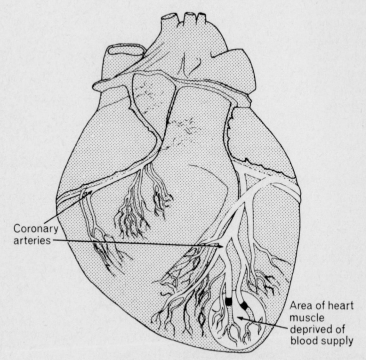

Coronary arteries

Area of heart muscle deprived of blood supply

FIG. 11.1. Blockage of two branches of the coronary artery

coronary thrombosis. Since diabetics do not take sugar, this is a help-ful step in reducing the risk of coronary thrombosis. Fat in the diet is also open to suspicion as a cause of coronary disease. It has been dem-onstrated that animal fats cause a rise in the cholesterol normally present in the blood and since a high cholesterol is related to the depo-sition of fat in the vessel wall, it seems reasonable in these circum-stances to reduce the amount of animal fat and butter in the diet. Fortunately, many vegetable fats such as corn oil contain a form of fat which in no way disposes to a rise in cholesterol, indeed the contrary is true. Consequently, many diets have been evolved which cut out butter, cream and animal fats from the diet entirely and substitute specially prepared oils prepared from vegetables. This diet is expensive, unpalatable and difficult to organize. At present, the evi-dence is not sufficiently strong to warrant disorganizing the whole of the household dietary routine on the dubious grounds that this might reduce the risks of coronary thrombosis in the years ahead.

There are other factors which dispose to the onset of coronary thrombosis which the diabetic can do much to avoid. Cigarette smok-ing is known to be a dangerous habit which carries with it a high mor-tality rate, partly due to its propensity to induce lung cancer. However, it has been convincingly demonstrated that cigarette smok-ing also disposes to coronary thrombosis and the incidence of coron-ary disease in men of 50 who smoke cigarettes heavily is twice as high as in those who do not smoke at all. Under these circumstances, it is plainly folly for diabetic patients to smoke cigarettes and this habit should be discontinued. Obesity is a further factor which disposes to coronary disease and since obesity is also deleterious as far as the dia-betes is concerned, it can only be stressed that every diabetic should try to maintain his weight at a normal level. Coronary thrombosis is much more liable to occur in those who lead a sedentary existence than in those who are more active. Bus conductors are less liable to coronary thrombosis than bus drivers, perhaps because the former use their legs much more. Here again, it behoves every diabetic patient to take as much regular physical exercise as he reasonably can and not to allow himself to become too sluggish and inert. Coronary thrombosis is also related to stress and strain. Men engaged in stress-ful occupations are more liable to develop thrombosis than those whose lives are on an even tenor and who carry less responsibility. It is always good advice to tell people not to worry, but this is advice much easier to give than to follow.

In summary then, although the diabetic is more liable to develop coronary thrombosis than the non-diabetic, he can considerably reduce these risks by keeping his weight to a normal level, by giving up smoking, by leading an active life, and by controlling his diabetes as carefully as he can.

FEET

Especially in elderly diabetics, there is a great need to take special care of the feet, since diabetes can affect the blood circulation and reduce sensation. Furthermore, the eyesight may be poor. Hence, the elderly diabetic may be divorced from his feet since he can neither feel them nor see them properly. Since the circulation is impaired, the feet are often cold and do not react well to changes of temperature. Furthermore, they are very liable to minor damage because sensation is impaired. Consequently even roughness in the shoe or sitting in front of too hot a fire can do serious damage without the patient being aware of it. Furthermore, since bacteria thrive when there is a lot of sugar in the blood, a small area of damage on the foot can quickly become septic. For these reasons, elderly patients must be particularly careful to examine their feet if they can or allow somebody else to do so at regular intervals if the eyesight is impaired. There is no doubt that a visit to the chiropodist from time to time is a sensible investment.

The feet should be washed daily in warm water, using a mild form of toilet soap. The skin should be dried carefully particularly between the toes and it is better to dab them with a soft towel without rubbing too much. When toenails need cutting, it is best to do this after the bath when the nail is softer. The edge should follow the shape of the end of the toe. It is a mistake to cut the nails too short and to try to cut into the corners of the nails. Using a sharp instrument to clean the nail grooves can lead to damage and should be avoided.

If the skin is very dry, it is a good practice to apply a little cream containing lanolin after bathing the feet. Closely packed or overlapping toes can be separated with wisps of lambswool but this must not encircle the toe as this may constrict the circulation.

It is most important to avoid getting into an overheated bath and it pays to test the temperature of the bath by using the hands or the elbow, which are more likely to be sensitive than the feet. When the feet are cold, it is most important to avoid sitting too close to heaters or fires. It is a good idea to warm the bed at night with hot water bottles or an elctric blanket, but the hot water bottle must be removed and the blanket switched off before getting into the bed. Loose fitting thick woollen bed socks are very helpful.

Shoes and socks must be comfortable and loose fitting. It is best to place the hands in the shoe before putting it on since the hands may note stones or nails that the insensitive foot may not detect. Women should not use tight garters which can only impair the circulation. Certainly, females should avoid wearing shoes with pointed toes and high heels since these constrict the circulation in the toes.

Finally, it is dangerous to try oneself to cut corns, callosities and ingrowing toenails. These minor ailments are much better treated by a chiropodist who knows how to avoid damaging the areas. Even a minor abrasion can lead to serious damage when the circulation is impaired with the foot insensitive and the sugar in the blood high. Minor cuts and abrasions should be covered with clean or sterile gauze and lightly bandaged. It is most important that damaged areas should be inspected regularly to ensure that they are healing cleanly.

It is as well to seek advice if there is any prominent colour change in the toes or feet, if there are any septic areas on the foot or if there is any undue pain or swelling in the feet. It is important that diabetics should understand that their feeling of pain or heat or cold may be impaired and only regular inspection can reveal damage to the feet which might otherwise pass unnoticed. Even apparently trivial wounds and injuries if not treated carefully may lead to serious complications and even gangrene. With good control of the diabetes, regular inspection and common sense, serious danger to the feet can nearly always be avoided. Prevention is better than cure.

EYES

Many diabetic patients realize that diabetes can affect the eyesight and often have unexpressed fears in this direction. It can be said at the outset that although diabetes can damage the eyes, it is exceptional for it to do so in any way which is liable seriously to disturb the vision. Blindness can be caused by diabetes but the risks of this happening are so slight that no diabetic should go through life fearing something which will never happen in the vast majority of diabetic patients. Many of the visual disturbances that occur in diabetes also occur very frequently in those without this ailment. Much thought and research has gone on and is going on into the cause and prevention of damage to the eyes in diabetes.

The eye is basically an apparatus which concentrates light on the retina, a very sensitive area carrying images to the brain for necessary interpretation. The light which reaches the eye is concentrated on the retina by a lens, just as the lens of a camera focuses the light on the film. This lens can be altered in size by muscles which cause it to narrow or broaden and so enable us to focus sometimes on objects nearby and sometimes on objects at a distance. The lens is protected from excessive light by the iris which lies in front of the lens and acts as a screen. The iris is pigmented usually green, blue or brown (which gives the eye its characteristic colour) and is impermeable to light. In strong light the iris narrows and permits only a small amount of light to pass through the lens, while in semi-darkness the iris opens very wide to allow as much light as possible to pass through the lens.

The retina itself consists of special nerve cells highly sensitive to light, rather like photo-electric cells. The impulses from these cells are carried via the optic nerve through the back of the eye to areas of the

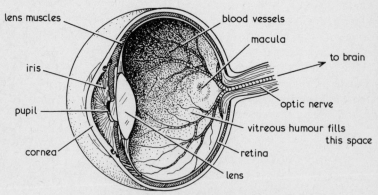

FIG. 11.2. Diagrammatic section through the eyeball

brain particularly devoted to the interpretation of images received from the retina. Thus in reading this page, light from the print is transmitted through the lens to the retina and from the retina to the occipital lobes of the brain. Here the meaning of the symbols is interpreted and sorted out for necessary action just as a computer receives messages for storage and action.

The retina can be inspected by an instrument known as the ophthalmoscope. This is a system of lenses illuminated by a strong light which enables the physician to peer through the lens of the eye into the retina. The retina appears as a red area with small blood vessels coursing across it. These blood vessels carry the essential blood supply to the nerve cells of the retina and so are of vital importance for the proper nourishment and oxygenation of the retina. The arteries carry fresh blood to the nerve cells while the veins return blood to the heart after oxygen and nutriments have been absorbed. Both arteries and veins can be seen with the ophthalmoscope and provide vital information to the physician as to the state of the arteries in general. He can look for evidence of arteriosclerosis because in these circumstances the arteries are thickened, narrowed and tortuous. The ophthalmoscope offers a unique opportunity of inspecting small arteries not otherwise available to the human eye except at surgical operation. Needless to say, the retina is only visible if the lens itself is transparent and consequently when a cataract exists the retina cannot be visualized.

The interior of the eye contains a jelly-like fluid called the vitreous humour which fills the eyeball and supports the retina. The composition of the vitreous humour is influenced by the state of the blood and by the amount of sugar in it. When the amount of sugar rises in the blood, the sugar in the vitreous humour increases at the same time and leads to changes of refraction in the light passing from the lens to the retina.

Disturbances of vision in diabetes can be due to many different causes, not all of them necessarily specific to diabetes itself.

Temporary disturbances of vision can occur due to changes in the blood sugar reflected in the vitreous humour. In the early stages of diabetes before diagnosis is made, the steadily increasing blood sugar levels cause a change of refraction in the eye and patients often go to the optician for new glasses. This change of vision is very gradual and usually unnoticed. However, when treatment is instituted and the blood sugars somewhat rapidly restored to normal, there is often a noticeable blurring of vision. In fact, this simply means that the state of the vitreous humour is being restored to normal and it is therefore unwise for a newly diagnosed and treated diabetic patient to get a change of glasses until he is quite sure that the diabetes has been stabilized. A temporary change in vision is often observed with the onset of hypoglycaemia, due to excessive action of insulin. In this case, it is the deprivation of sugar in the vitreous humour which leads to blurring of vision and this is a common warning symptom of hypoglycaemia. It is soon put to right when sugar is taken. In diabetics prone to migraine hypoglycaemia can sometimes precipitate an attack with characteristic flashes of light or zigzag visual patterns.

Cataracts are very common in elderly patients in general but diabetes is probably an exacerbating factor since patients with diabetes are prone to develop cataracts at a rather younger age than those with normal blood sugars. A cataract is due to clouding of the lens. We are not quite sure what causes this change of structure in the lens but thick fibres form in the lens which ultimately becomes entirely opaque to light. Indeed, it is often easily apparent on ordinary examination of the eye when the cataract appears as a white area in the centre of the iris. The usual early symptoms of cataract formation are blurring of vision and loss of visual definition, particularly troublesome in poor light. It becomes increasingly difficult to read and to see the television screen. It is surprising and disappointing that many people allow this state of affairs to occur and develop without seeking medical advice, because operative procedure can make such a vast difference. When the lens has become entirely opaque, its removal is not a difficult operation in skilled hands. Once the damaged lens has been removed, light can once again reach the retina. However, the ability to focus, normally the main function of the lens, is permanently lost after cataract extraction and so glasses must be used for reading and for long-distance vision. This is a minor disadvantage.

The retina itself can be damaged in diabetes though the exact nature and cause of this disorder is not fully understood. In the early stages, the veins of the retina can be seen to be somewhat enlarged and irregular. Small dots can be observed through the ophthalmoscope and we now know that these represent small bulges or microaneurysms in the wall of the capillaries which join the arteries to the veins. These microaneurysms represent a weakness of the vessel wall and may actually rupture with spillage of blood into the retina. Local haemorrhages formed in this way can be seen with the ophthalmoscope as small rounded areas in the retina. In a severe case, haemorrhages might be frequent and may extend into the vitreous humour with disturbance of vision. There is one area of the retina which is most sensitive to vision. This area is known as the macula and if the macula is involved in a haemorrhage, vision can be seriously impaired. In addition to haemorrhages, white patches known as exudates can sometimes be seen in the diabetic retina. These probably represent degenerated areas of the retina inadequately provided with a blood supply from the capillaries. The exudates can become so extensive as to ultimately interfere with visual acuity. In a grossly severe case, haemorrhages and exudates can together extinguish vision altogether and blindness ensues. Happily, progressive cases of this kind are rare.

Changes in the retina are often observed after diabetes has been present for more than fifteen or twenty years. Small microaneurysms, haemorrhages and exudates may be seen, but these may have no effect on the patient's vision whatsoever. These changes are related to some extent to the control of the diabetes, in that they appear more commonly in patients whose blood sugars are nearly always greatly elevated and whose dietary habits are irregular. Consequently, physicians who undertake the care of diabetic patients will always stress the need for regularity of diet and insulin in the hope of reducing the risks of degenerative changes in the retina. Nevertheless, it must be said in honesty that diabetic control is not the only factor responsible for retinal disorders. They sometimes occur in patients with very mild diabetes and blood sugars scarcely elevated above normal. It is clear that there are factors occurring in diabetes, other than the raised blood sugar, which contribute to the changes taking place in the retina. A vast amount of research has been undertaken and is being undertaken to elucidate the cause and prevention of these retinal disorders and there is little doubt that as time goes on more effective methods will become available to prevent and treat this retinal damage. It is sometimes asked whether the type of treatment bears any relation to the onset of retinal changes but so far there is no evidence that either tablets or insulin has any preferential effect on the progress of these disorders.

Although good diabetic control isn't the only factor involved in the development of damage to the retina in diabetes, there is no doubt at all that diabetics who look after themselves carefully and try to keep their blood sugars as near normal as possible are much less likely to ever develop retinal changes. It is for this reason that stress is made on the need to keep fit in general and to look after the diabetes in particular, with regular diet and regular control of the blood sugar. However, direct treatment of the retina has become available in recent years and it is incumbent on every diabetic patient to have his eyes inspected regularly so that the first sign of trouble can be detected and treated if necessary. This new approach is known as photocoagulation.

Photocoagulation is a form of treatment in which an intense laser beam of light is thrown on areas of the retina in which damage has occurred. The laser beam cauterises the small microaneurysms and prevents the bleeding which is responsible for the damage. Two sources of light are used for photocoagulation. One is the xenon arc and the other the argon laser. They act rather like a magnifying glass does when it concentrates the rays of the sun to burn a piece of paper. Of course, the apparatus is expensive and a skilled ophthalmic surgeon is needed to use it. Nevertheless, the treatment is painless and has proved to be very effective in preventing deterioration in eyes already damaged by diabetic retinal changes. Photocoagulation has become a powerful tool in the prevention of loss of vision from diabetes.

When exudates are seen in the retina, a low fat diet and clofibrate tablets may be tried. This routine lowers the cholesterol in the blood and since the exudates contain cholesterol-like substances, may lead to a marked diminution in the extent of the exudates. Unfortunately, the areas of retina in which exudates appear are already damaged so that visual acuity may not noticeably improve even though the exudates disappear.

Blindness and loss of vision are both comparatively rare occurrences in diabetes but since diabetes is such a common disorder, sufficient numbers of patients are faced with this problem to warrant programmes of training and the setting up of special establishments to deal with the problem. When the eyesight is deteriorating, considerable adjustment of training and attitude may become necessary.

It is often best to be trained to read Braille before vision has been lost absolutely since learning Braille is immeasurably easier when some vision still exists.

It cannot be too strongly stressed that visual disturbance of this severity is infrequent and a recent estimation suggests that only three of every thousand unaffected eyes develop serious visual loss due to diabetes each year. Nevertheless, research is continuing in an endeavour to overcome this serious problem.

NEURITIS AND RENAL INFECTION

Diabetes can affect the nerves of the legs and symptoms may appear when the blood sugar has been allowed to remain elevated for too long. These symptoms are those of tingling in the extremities, sometimes associated with muscle cramps, numbness and pain. As a rule these features abate when the diabetes is controlled. But sometimes neuritis can occur even in a well-controlled case, suggesting factors other than an elevated level of blood sugar may be responsible.

Renal infection is more common in diabetics and may give rise to frequency of passing water, sometimes associated with burning discomfort. This infection of the urinary tract may be in the bladder (cystitis) or in the kidney (pyelitis). The diagnosis can be confirmed by collecting a specimen of urine and culturing it to see if bacteria are present. In addition examination under the microscope may reveal the presence of white cells, called out in order to deal with a bacterial infection and not normally present in the urine. If bacteria and white cells are found, appropriate antibiotic treatment should be given. It is important to treat these conditions since if they are allowed to continue over the years, chronic damage to the kidneys may ensue. Hence it is wise for the diabetic patient to report infections of this type to the doctor who can assess whether further investigation is necessary.

SEXUAL FUNCTION

There are three aspects of sexual function in the male that may be impaired, in diabetics as in non-diabetics, and because the cause of the impairment may often be emotional rather than organic, it is as well to understand fully what is involved. The three aspects of sexual function to be considered are libido, potency and fertility and any one of these may be disordered.

By libido we mean the natural sexual desire that a man feels for the opposite sex and the arousal of sexual interest by being near the female. In any constitutional illness, sex drive is lost. In the early stages of diabetes, before treatment has been instituted, there is a general loss of energy and interest, and this loss includes libido. The male sex drive is powered by sex hormones called androgens, produced by special cells in the testicles and by the adrenal glands situated above the kidneys. Depression of mood or general ill health from any cause leads to suppression of androgen production and consequent falling off of sex interest. Once the general health is restored by proper treatment, normal sexual desire soon returns.

Potency in the male means the ability to maintain an erection during sexual intercourse. Apart from loss of libido already mentioned, the commonest cause of loss of potency is emotional insecurity. Failure of erection can occur from fear of failure to perform the sex act properly, from lack of confidence or general anxiety. Usually with love and understanding from the female, this cause of impotency can be overcome. Characteristically, the male with emotional impotency will find he has a normal erection on waking in the morning, thus proving that the physical mechanism is not at fault when not inhibited by nervousness or stress. The mechanism of erection is partly under control of the nerve fibres supplying the male organ (penis) and when diabetes has been present for many years (usually more than 20 years) in some cases these nerves can be affected. In this situation, loss of potency is due to neuritis and not to emotional causes.

By fertility we mean the ability to produce live sperm from the testicle and this ability is unimpaired in diabetes. Even when impotency has occurred with inability to maintain an erection, ejaculation of live sperm will still be possible.

With well-controlled diabetes, libido, potency and fertility should all be normal. Only in those men who have had diabetes for many years is there a liability to neuritis which can occasionally lead to loss of potency.

In the female with diabetes, sexual function is unimpaired. The female diabetic is as likely to conceive as the non-diabetic and, as has been discussed, has every reason to expect a healthy baby. Young girls who develop diabetes may find that the menstrual periods come on rather later than average but this is of no significance.

12

SOME APPROPRIATE DIETS

Reducing diets on page 135 are for patients who are overweight; if weight is reduced, no other treatment for diabetes may be necessary.

Diets on pages 136–7 are mainly for patients who are having tablet treatment. The diet continues to be of prime importance and if it is not adhered to the tablets may lose their effect.

The remaining diets are for patients taking insulin. Since insulin acts throughout the day, food must be taken at regular intervals as shown. It may be dangerous to be late for meals or to omit snack meals.

The diets are constructed using the commonest kinds of food. Lists of alternatives are given on pages 139–42, so that monotony can be avoided. It is possible to enjoy a varied and appetising diet, making use of the ordinary foods available in the shops, and avoiding any separate individual cooking.

In all the diets, the lunch and supper meals are interchangeable, and the supper meal may be taken as a packed lunch if more convenient.

HOUSEHOLD MEASURES

With a little practice and by memorising these few handy measures, patients should be able to control their own dietary intake, both at home and when eating out, without constant use of weighing scales.

1 oz bread	1 whole thin slice from a large cut loaf, or 1¼ whole thin slices from a small loaf
¼ oz butter	Sufficient to cover thinly 1 oz bread
3 oz boiled potato	1 potato, the size of a large egg.

1 oz boiled rice, macaroni, spaghetti, etc.	1 tablespoonful, **not** heaped
3 oz lean meat	A large serving
2 oz cheese	A piece the size of a matchbox
Milk	Milk can be measured in small graduated measuring jug

$\frac{1}{3}$ pint = approx 1 breakfastcupful
$\frac{1}{4}$ pint = approx 1 teacupful

REDUCING DIETS

800 CALORIES
Approx 57 *g carbohydrate;* 62 *g protein;* 39 *g fat*

Breakfast (15 g carb)
Egg or alternative
Bread 1 oz , butter scraped off
Milk for tea – from **allowance**

Mid-morning (if required)
Bovril, etc., or dietetic fruit squash

Lunch (10 g carb)
Lean meat 3 oz
Green vegetables or salad
Fruit – one portion

Tea (15 g carb)
Bread 1 oz , butter scraped off
Salad, etc.
Milk for tea – from **allowance**

Supper (10 g carb)
Lean meat 3 oz
Green vegetables or salad
Fruit – one portion

Bedtime (if required)
Bovril, etc., or dietetic fruit squash

Daily allowance   Milk $\frac{1}{4}$ pint (7 g carb)   Butter scraping

1200 CALORIES
Approx 94 *g carbohydrate;* 62 *g protein;* 64 *g fat*

Breakfast (15 g carb)
Egg or alternative
Bread 1 oz , butter from allowance
Milk for tea – from allowance

Mid-morning
Milk for tea or coffee – from allowance

Lunch (25 g carb)
Lean meat 3 oz
Green vegetables
Boiled potatoes 3 oz
Fruit – one portion

Tea (15 g carb)
Bread 1 oz , butter from allowance
Salad, etc.
Milk for tea – from allowance

Supper (25 g carb)
Cheese 2 oz , or alternative
Green vegetables or salad
Bread 1 oz – butter from allowance
Fruit – one portion

Bedtime
Milk for tea or coffee – from allowance

Daily allowance   Milk $\frac{1}{2}$ pint   Butter $\frac{1}{2}$ oz

TABLET TREATMENT

1500 CALORIES

Approx 140 g carbohydrate; 68 g protein; 77 g fat

Breakfast (33 g carb)
Egg or alternative
Bread 2 oz
Butter ¼ oz
Milk for tea 2 oz

Tea (25 g carb)
Bread 1½ oz
Butter ¼ oz
Salad, etc.
Milk for tea 2 oz

Mid-morning (3 g carb)
Milk for tea or coffee 2 oz

Supper (35 g carb)
Cheese 2 oz , or alternative
Green vegetables or salad
Bread 1½ oz
Butter ¼ oz
Fruit – one portion
Milk for tea or coffee 2 oz

Lunch (37 g carb)
Lean meat 2 oz
Green vegetables
Boiled potatoes 3 oz
Milk pudding or alternative (see page 142)

Bedtime (7 g carb)
Milk for tea or coffee 5 oz

Daily allowance   Milk 1 pint   Butter ¾ oz

1800 CALORIES

Approx 178 g carbohydrate; 75 g protein; 95 g fat

Breakfast (42 g carb)
Egg or alternative
Cereal ½ oz
Bread 1½ oz
Butter ¼ oz
Milk for tea and cereal 5 oz

Tea (25 g carb)
Bread 1½ oz
Butter ¼ oz
Salad, etc.
Milk for tea 2 oz

Supper (43 g carb)
Cheese 2 oz , or alternative
Green vegetables or salad
Bread 2 oz
Butter ½ oz
Fruit – one portion
Milk for tea or coffee 2 oz

Mid-morning (5 g carb)
Milk for tea or coffee 3½ oz

Lunch (45 g carb)
Lean meat 2 oz
Green vegetables
Boiled potatoes 4 oz
Milk pudding or alternative (see page 142)

Bedtime (18 g carb)
Milk 5 oz
2 plain biscuits

2000 CALORIES

Approx 197 *g carbohydrate;* 80 *g protein;* 106 *g fat*

Breakfast (45 g carb)
Egg or alternative
Cereal ½ oz
Bread 1½ oz
Butter ¼ oz
Milk for tea and cereal 7 oz

Mid-morning (16 g carb)
Milk for tea or coffee 3½ oz
2 plain biscuits

Lunch (45 g carb)
Lean meat 2 oz
Green vegetables
Boiled potatoes 4 oz
Milk pudding or alternative (see page 142)

Tea (28 g carb)
Bread 1½ oz
Butter ¼ oz
Salad, etc.
Milk for tea 3½ oz

Supper (45 g carb)
Cheese 2 oz , or alternative
Green vegetables or salad
Bread 2 oz
Butter ½ oz
Fruit – one portion
Milk for tea or coffee 3½ oz

Bedtime (18 g carb)
Milk 5 oz
2 plain biscuits

2200 CALORIES

Approx 218 *g carbohydrate;* 84 *g protein;* 112 *g fat*

Breakfast (53 g carb)
Egg or alternative
Cereal ½ oz
Bread 2 oz
Butter ½ oz
Milk for tea and cereal 7 oz

Mid-morning (16 g carb)
Milk for tea or coffee 3½ oz
2 plain biscuits

Lunch (50 g carb)
Lean meat 2 oz
Green vegetables
Boiled potatoes 5 oz
Milk pudding or alternative (see page 142)

Tea (28 g carb)
Bread 1½ oz
Butter ¼ oz
Salad, etc.
Milk for tea 3½ oz

Supper (53 g carb)
Cheese 2 oz, or alternative
Green vegetables or salad
Bread 2½ oz
Butter ½ oz
Fruit – one portion
Milk for tea or coffee 3½ oz

Bedtime (18 g. carb.)
Milk 5 oz
2 plain biscuits

INSULIN TREATMENT

2500 CALORIES
Approx 250 g carbohydrate; 95 g protein; 126 g fat

Breakfast (60 g carb)
2 eggs or alternative
Cereal ½ oz
Bread 2½ oz
Butter ½ oz
Milk for tea and cereal 7 oz

Mid-morning (16 g carb)
Milk for tea or coffee 3½ oz
2 plain biscuits

Lunch (62 g carb)
Lean meat 2 oz
Green vegetables
Boiled potatoes 7 oz
Milk pudding or alternative (see page 142)

Tea (35 g carb)
Bread 2 oz
Butter ½ oz
Salad, etc.
Milk for tea 3½ oz

Supper (60 g carb)
Cheese 2 oz , or alternative
Green vegetables or salad
Bread 3 oz
Butter ½ oz
Fruit – one portion
Milk for tea or coffee 3½ oz

Bedtime (18 g carb)
Milk 5 oz
2 plain biscuits

2800 CALORIES
Approx 279 g carbohydrate; 100 g protein; 144 g fat

Breakfast (68 g carb)
2 eggs or alternative
Cereal ½ oz
Bread 3 oz
Butter ½ oz
Milk for tea and cereal 7 oz

Mid-morning (16 g carb)
Milk for tea or coffee 3½ oz
2 plain biscuits

Lunch (68 g carb)
Lean meat 2 oz
Green vegetables
Boiled potatoes 8 oz
Milk pudding or alternative (see page 142)

Tea (35 g carb)
Bread 2 oz
Butter ½ oz
Salad, etc
Milk for tea 3½ oz

Supper (68 g carb)
Cheese 2 oz , or alternative
Green vegetables or salad
Bread 3½ oz
Butter ¾ oz
Fruit – one portion
Milk for tea or coffee 3½ oz

Bedtime (26 g carb)
Milk 7 oz
3 plain biscuits
Butter ¼ oz

ALTERNATIVES

CARBOHYDRATE

Carbohydrate foods are of great importance in the treatment of diabetes since they are mainly converted to sugar soon after being eaten. Patients should learn the carbohydrate values of foods and should be particularly careful not to exceed their allowance. Common carbohydrate foods are bread, biscuits, potatoes, rice, cereals and fruit.

The quality of carbohydrate food is just as important as the quantity. Unnatural concentrated foods made with sugar and white flour are quickly converted to glucose and absorbed straight into the blood. Natural carbohydrate foods containing a high fibre content are broken down more slowly in the bowel (see page 3) and so do not cause a rapid rise in the blood sugar. Wholemeal bread, wholewheat flour and brown rice are preferable to white bread, white flour and polished rice. Cakes and biscuits should be made from wholewheat flour, oatmeal or rolled oats with dried fruits and nuts. Breakfast cereals should consist of whole wheat or oats including such brands as All-Bran, Weetabix, Shredded Wheat and porridge oats. If the bowels are constipated, a tablespoon of natural or unprocessed bran can be mixed with the breakfast cereal. Fresh fruit, vegetables and salads are valuable in that they provide natural dietary fibre.

Carbohydrate exchanges ($= 10$ g. carb.)

$\frac{2}{3}$ oz. bread ($= \frac{2}{3}$ thin slice from a large cut loaf) may be replaced by any of the following:

$\frac{1}{2}$ oz plain biscuits
$\frac{1}{2}$ oz Ryvita
$\frac{1}{2}$ oz breakfast cereal
$\frac{1}{2}$ oz rice, macaroni, spaghetti, sago, semolina (raw weight), flour
2 oz boiled potatoes, or 1 oz chips, or $1\frac{1}{2}$ oz roast potatoes

2 oz boiled haricot or butter beans, lentils or split peas, boiled
2 oz tinned peas or baked beans
3 oz boiled parsnips
$3\frac{1}{2}$ oz boiled beetroot
1 oz chestnuts
(1 portion of fruit (as below)

Fruit portions (one portion = 10 g carb)

Note. Each portion is equal in carbohydrate value to $\frac{2}{3}$oz bread.

Apples	4 oz	= 1 dessert
Stewed apples	5 oz	= large helping
Apricots (dried, stewed)	2½ oz	= 3 or 4
Bananas (no skins)	2 oz	= 1 small or ½ large
Blackcurrants, blackberries	8 oz	= moderate helping
Cherries (raw with stones)	3 oz	= 6–8
Grapes	2½ oz	= 6–8
Greengages (raw with stones)	3 oz	= 3–4
Melon	7 oz	= large helping
Oranges (no skins)	4 oz	= 1 dessert
Fresh orange juice	4 oz	
Peaches (fresh with stones)	5 oz	= 1 dessert
Pear	5 oz	= 1 dessert
Pineapple (fresh)	3 oz	= 1 small slice
Plums (Victoria, whole)	4 oz	= small helping
Stewed plums	8 oz	= large helping
Prunes (dried, stewed)	2 oz	= 3 or 4
Strawberries, raspberries	6 oz	= small helping
Tangerines (no skins)	4 oz	= 2 small

*Dairy products** (= 10 g carb)

Milk   7 oz

Milk, evaporated, unsweetened 3 oz   Ice cream (plain)   2 oz

Note. The sign * indicates that these values are for carbohydrate content only. In view of the high protein and fat content of milk and ice cream, the calorie value of the diet is considerably increased when these are included.

Foods with a very high carbohydrate content (which should be avoided)

Sugar, glucose
Jam, marmalade, honey, etc.
Sweets, chocolate, ice cream
Cakes, pastries, sweet biscuits, puddings made with flour
Thickened soups, sauces and gravies
Sweet wines and soft drinks
Fruit tinned in syrup

Extras allowed (the following may be taken freely)

Green vegetables and salads
Stewed rhubarb or stewed gooseberries
½ grapefruit
Bovril, Oxo, Marmite, clear soup without thickening or noodles
Black tea or coffee (not coffee essence)
Sugarless fruit squashes, soda water, water

Meat and fish pastes in moderate amounts
Vinegar, clear vinegar pickles, sharp sauces, e.g. Worcester
Lemon juice   2½ oz
Flavouring and seasoning, e.g. curry powder, herbs, spices
Saccharine or saxin for sweetening
Nuts in moderate amounts (except chestnuts – see *carbohydrate exchanges*)
Table jellies made from unsweetened jelly crystals, with saccharine added to taste,
    or from sugarless fruit squash and gelatine

HIGH FIBRE DIET

Especially where constipation is troublesome, the amount of fibre in the diet should be
increased. The high fibre diet is beneficial in diabetes because it delays the absorption
of sugar formed from carbohydrate.

Bread	Replace white or brown breads by wholemeal breads made from whole wheat or whole rye
Flour	Use 100% extraction wholemeal flour.
Cakes and biscuits	Made with wholemeal flour, oatmeal or rolled oats, dried fruit and nuts. Use whole grain crispbreads (e.g. Ryvita).
Cereals	All-Bran, Shredded Wheat, Weetabix, Puffed Wheat, porridge oats, muesli.
Fruit, nuts, vegetables, salads	Eat raw where possible, e.g. in the form of coleslaw (shredded cabbage, grated apple, carrots and onions, with seasoning and nuts, combined with yoghurt).

PROTEIN

The main foods containing protein are: meat, poultry, offal, fish,
cheese and eggs. When arranging alternative menus it is important
to include as much of these foods as is used in the basic diets.

(*a*) **Breakfast alternatives**
Instead of 1 egg you may have:
1 rasher (1 oz) bacon   1 small piece (3 oz) smoked haddock
1 slice (1 oz) cold ham   1 small kipper (3 oz.)

(*b*) **Lunch alternatives**
Instead of 2 oz lean meat (an average helping) you may have:
2 oz poultry or rabbit   3 oz herring (1 small one)
2 oz liver or kidney, or other offal   2 oz cheese
4 oz white fish (one medium plaice   2 eggs
    fillet)

(*c*) **Supper alternatives**

Instead of 2 oz cheese you may have:

2 oz lean meat or bacon	2 eggs
2 oz sardines or tinned salmon, drained of oil	4 oz white fish, herring, or baked kipper

Butter, fats and cream

Margarine, butter, lard, meat fat, dripping, and olive oil all have the same calorie value and may be substituted for each other in equal amounts. They have no carbohydrate or protein value.

    Cream (double) contains half the calorie value of butter or margarine

MILK PUDDINGS (containing 20 g carbohydrate each) (as well as variable amounts of protein and fat)

The milk pudding in the diets should be made with:

> 7 oz ($\frac{1}{3}$ pint) milk
> $\frac{1}{2}$ oz rice, semolina, sago, etc.
> Saccharine to taste, if required

Some alternatives to this type of pudding are:

1. **Fruit and Custard**
One portion of stewed fruit (see list) with custard made from $\frac{1}{4}$ pint milk and $\frac{1}{4}$ oz custard powder.

2. **Fruit and Egg Custard**
One portion of stewed fruit (see list) with egg custard made from 7 oz milk (1 glass) and one egg.

3. **Bread and Butter Pudding**
5 oz. milk, $\frac{1}{2}$ an egg, $\frac{1}{3}$ oz bread, knob of butter and $\frac{1}{2}$ oz sultanas, baked in a dish surrounded by water in a moderate oven for about 45 minutes.

4. **Banana Custard**
2 oz. banana, $3\frac{1}{2}$ oz milk and $\frac{1}{4}$ oz custard powder. Slice banana into dish; make custard, pour on top, taking care to cover all fruit. Allow to set.

5. **Biscuits and Cheese**
Three water or four cracker biscuits, with $\frac{1}{4}$ oz butter and 1 oz cheese.

6. **Biscuits and Cheese with Fruit**
Two cracker biscuits, with $\frac{1}{4}$ oz butter, 1 oz cheese and one portion fruit (see list).

ALCOHOLIC BEVERAGES

Drink	Carbohydrate (g)	Calories
Bottled stout, ½ pint	12	100
Extra stout, ½ pint	6	110
Draught ale, mild, ½ pint	5	70
Strong ale, ½ pint	17	210
Cider, sweet, ½ pint	12	120
Cider, vintage, ½ pint	20	280
Cider, dry, ½ pint	8	100
Sherry, sweet, 1½ oz	3	57
Sherry, dry, 1½ oz	0.5	50
Champagne, glass, 5 oz	2	105
Graves, goblet, 6⅔ oz	6	140
Sauternes, goblet, 6⅔ oz	11	170
Beaujolais, goblet, 6⅔ oz	0.5	126
Spirits, 70% proof, gin, whisky, rum, etc., 1 oz	—	63

ADVICE

(FOR INSULIN PATIENTS ONLY)

IF YOU ARE TAKEN ILL

with influenza, sore throat, diarrhoea, or any other complaint which makes it difficult to take your usual diet

take your usual insulin at the usual time; the insulin must never be stopped;

take a tablespoonful of sugar in fruit squash or tea instead of the usual meal that is missed, and repeat this until you are able to take food;

call in your family doctor, especially if there is persistent vomiting.

IF YOU HAVE A REACTION

and feel sweaty, tremulous, or queer at any time, take two lumps of sugar. Never be late with your meals or miss your snacks. Always carry sugar with you.

CARE OF YOUR SYRINGE

1. Keep your syringe and needle in a spirit container or on a piece of lint and cover them with spirit.

2. Wash your hands before using the syringe and needle. See that no spirit is left in them before drawing up the insulin.

Cleanse the top of the insulin bottles with gauze dipped in spirit, and use the same gauze to cleanse the skin where you will inject.

3. Vary the site of injection each day. Do not push the needle more than half-way to avoid the risk of breaking it while injecting.

4. Disposable plastic syringes are available and are particularly useful when on holiday.

WHEN TO TEST YOUR URINE

1. Empty bladder on waking. Just before breakfast, pass another specimen and keep for testing.

2. Empty bladder in middle of morning. Just before the midday meal, pass another specimen and keep for testing.

3. Empty bladder in the middle of the afternoon. Just before the evening meal, pass another specimen and keep for testing.

4. Empty bladder after the evening meal. Just before going to bed, pass another specimen and keep for testing.

Of course, it is not suggested that the urine should be tested four times a day, every day: but these are the times most valuable in indicating whether the insulin dose needs adjustment (see page 80).

13

RESEARCH PROBLEMS

❧

Despite great advances in our understanding and treatment of diabetes, many aspects of this ailment remain entirely enigmatic. We are still ignorant as to the cause of diabetes and although present treatment allows most diabetics to lead full and healthy lives, in some we are unable to prevent the onset of disabling complications. Consequently, a great deal of research is conducted in medical and scientific centres, particularly in Europe and America, resulting in numerous scientific conferences and the publication annually of many thousands of scientific papers. The British Diabetic Association, founded in 1934 under the presidency of H. G. Wells (himself a diabetic), has done a great deal to foster research and has set up five research groups in this country to investigate various problems. Scientific meetings are held twice a year when progress in research investigations is presented and discussed. Some of the problems in our understanding of diabetes have already been mentioned in the text and what follows is designed to explain the sort of research that is being undertaken to clarify and improve our understanding and treatment of diabetes.

1. EXPERIMENTAL DIABETES

Much of our understanding of human diabetes is based on experiments on animals. Banting's original elucidation of the source of isolation of insulin followed his work on dogs. In 1935, Young demonstrated that a dog given repeated injections of pituitary extract ultimately developed diabetes, thus demonstrating the interplay of insulin with other hormones. Although diabetes occurs naturally in the animal kingdom, and indeed many pets are kept alive by insulin, from the viewpoint of the researcher more reliable methods must be found of obtaining diabetic animals. Several laboratory techniques are now available.

1. *Pancreatectomy* Surgical removal of the pancreas was originally performed by Mirkowski in 1889. This method is time-consuming, difficult to perform in many species, and disturbs the digestive processes.

2. *Alloxan* is a substance chemically related to uric acid, and uric acid appears as a normal product of protein metabolism in man. Alloxan itself has never been found in man in health or in diabetes but in 1943 experimenters established that when injected into the rabbit, alloxan led to a selective destruction of the islet cells of the pancreas and thus the development of diabetes. Alloxan has toxic effects on the kidney as well but for many years alloxan-diabetic animals have been used when the effect of new treatments or investigations has had to be assessed.

3. *Streptozotocin* is a derivative of the antibiotics and by chance has been found to depress the action of the islet cells of the pancreas. Unlike alloxan, it appears to be non-toxic to most species and the degee of islet cell depression is commensurate with the dosage used. In other words, small doses of streptozotocin lead to the mild type of diabetes seen in maturity-onset diabetes in man, while larger doses lead to the more severe type of diabetes seen in young people with high blood sugars and ketosis. Clearly, an experimental model of this type offers opportunities of investigation into the disorders of biochemistry leading to the production of ketosis and the onset of coma.

4. *The thiazide group of drugs* are powerful diuretics, much used in the treatment of congestive heart failure to eliminate (via the kidneys) the excessive fluid retained in the failing circulation. It began to be observed about 1960 that many patients under treatment with thiazides developed sugar in the urine and animal experimental work soon demonstrated that these drugs inhibited the release of insulin from the islet cells. Some of these compounds were more prone to produce diabetes than others and further work led to the isolation of diazoxide. This drug now has a place in the treatment of patients who produce too much insulin from a tumour of the islet cells.

5. Although insulin obtained from different animals may have the effect of lowering the blood sugar in all of them, in fact the structure of insulin is slightly different in each species. For example, of 51 amino-acids which comprise the insulin molecule, human insulin differs in three of them from bovine insulin. Nevertheless, so subtle is the body's ability to detect foreign material that the injection of bovine insulin into man leads to the formation of antibodies, not sufficiently strong to obstruct the effect of the injected insulin in most cases. However, this principle has been utilized in experimental work. Guinea pigs injected with ox insulin develop high quantities of antibodies in their serum: injections of this antiserum into mice block the action of insulin and render the mice diabetic. Similar techniques have been used in other species and have provided valuable information on the development of degenerative changes that can occur in diabetes.

2. ELECTRON MICROSCOPY

In the electron microscope the energy source is a beam of electrons emitted from a heated tungsten cathode and directed through a circular aperture in the anode. Beneath the anode are placed a series of magnetic fields. In terms of an ordinary microscope, the electron beam can be likened to the beam of light and the magnetic fields to the lenses which focus on the object. On passing through the specimen, usually a very thin section of tissue, some electrons are absorbed while others are diffracted. The transmitted electrons are ultimately focused to produce an image which is enlarged and projected on to a fluorescent screen. The observer can scan the specimen on the screen and permanent photographs of relevant material can be taken by a camera placed within the microscope. This technique has enabled cells and tissues to be studied in detail previously unattainable.

The factors which control the formation, storage and release of insulin are of fundamental importance in our understanding of diabetes and the use of the electron microscope has enabled us to study the islet cells of the pancreas in considerable detail. Granules of insulin can be seen to form within the beta cells, migrate to the cell boundary, and then discharge into the capillaries. Glucose and the sulphonylureas demonstrably stimulate this process, though how they do so is unknown. The insulin granules must find their way through several structures before entering the bloodstream and there is evidence that one of these structures, the basement membrane of the vessel wall, may be abnormally thickened in diabetes. If this were so, the impoverishment of insulin supply in diabetes could be secondary to changes in the capillary walls, a theory much debated and under investigation. Examination of other tissues, notably the kidney, has shown that thickening of the basement membrane is not restricted to the pancreas. Study of the kidney in diabetes has been facilitated by the needle biopsy, a safe technique in which a minute portion of kidney is removed by a special needle and can then be examined under the electron microscope. Work on these lines has been undertaken on the kidney glomerulus, which filters urine from the blood and has revealed thickening of the basement membrane of its surrounding blood capillaries. Two explanations are possible. The first, that the thickened lining of the capillaries is due to diabetes, perhaps caused by the raised blood sugar. The second, that the changes seen in the basement membrane are due to some basic metabolic disorder responsible also for a delay in insulin release. Clearly these studies open new fields of investigation.

3. STRUCTURE OF INSULIN

The complete structure of insulin was worked out by Sanger in 1955. He used various enzymes to break down ox insulin into smaller groups of amino-acids. These were then analysed and their structural sequence established. Insulin consists of two amino-acid chains of unequal length, the A chain containing 21 amino-acids and the B chain 30. The two chains are linked by disulphide bridges. Although insulin from different species follows the same general plan in structure, differences exist in certain of the amino-acid sequences, particularly in the A chain. These variations are reflected in the shape of the insulin granules seen under the electron microscope which show different characteristics for different animals. Since the granules are too large to represent single molecules of insulin, the amino-acid sequence must in some way influence the arrangement of the molecules in the granules.

The structure of insulin has recently been synthesized from blocks of amino-acids by Katsoyannis and other workers, thus confirming its structure beyond question and opening the way for the preparation of effective modifications of insulin. The great hope is that a form of insulin could be prepared impervious to the digestive juices which could be given by mouth. Some semi-synthetic insulins have been prepared and these have been shown to supress the blood sugar levels in experimental animals. Whether or not this form of insulin will have clinical application remains to be seen and is the subject of active research.

In 1967 Steiner was investigating the biosynthesis of insulin in human islet cell tumour slices. The tumour, which had been successfully removed at operation, produced vast quantities of insulin and had caused repeated hypoglycaemic attacks in the patient before its detection and removal. Amino-acids were rendered radioactive to enable their easy detection, and were fed into the tumour. The tumour slices successfully synthesized radioactive insulin from the amino-acids. What was puzzling was that radioactive molecules larger than insulin first appeared with some of the properties of insulin though unable to reduce blood sugars. Steiner deduced that this larger molecule, which he named pro-insulin, was a precursor of insulin. It contained 84 amino-acids including the 21 A chain sequence, the 30 B chain sequence, and a connecting chain of 33 amino-acids. When treated with suitable enzymes, the connecting chain detached, leaving the normal insulin molecule. This brilliant investigation suggested the possibility that diabetes could result because an enzyme was missing which failed to convert the inactive pro-insulin to active insulin. However, so far studies in diabetics have failed to demonstrate a high proportion of pro-insulin to fit in with this thesis.

4. THE ARTIFICIAL PANCREAS AND TRANSPLANTATION

The artificial pancreas is an experimental apparatus which relies on an insulin pump and a glucose analyser, coupled to a computer. By inserting a catheter into the vein of a diabetic subject, blood is constantly drawn off for regular estimation of blood sugar levels. The results are transmitted to the computer which then instructs the insulin pump as to how much insulin to inject. By this means, subjects with diabetes have had their blood sugars kept at a normal level for several days. Needless to say, the apparatus is bulky and is certainly not transportable as yet. Nevertheless, methods have already been worked out for a simpler method of estimating the blood sugar levels and for simpler methods of giving insulin at a steady rate. Very fine filamentous tubes have been inserted under the skin and maintained there without discomfort for several days. A small pump apparatus can be attached to the tube, delivering insulin at a steady rate in accordance with blood sugar changes. This type of apparatus may be further refined and may become a practicable possibility in the future, though as yet many difficulties have to be overcome.

Healthy pancreas glands have been removed from subjects who have recently died and whose relatives have agreed to make these glands available to severe long-standing diabetics. Of course, the body tends to reject foreign material and it is only in a small proportion of cases that a good match can be found between an available pancreas gland and the diabetic subject needing the transplant. However, this operation has now been done in several cases, though only with moderate success. In most cases, after a variable amount of time, perhaps a year or so, the foreign pancreas is either rejected or fails to function properly. The technique is therefore not a practical possibility, though it is still being done in diabetics who have serious kidney disease and can have both a renal and pancreatic transplant at the same time.

Much more interesting is the possibility of transplanting not the whole pancreas glands, but merely the islet cells which produce insulin. The islet cells of Langerhans occupy only a small part of the pancreatic gland but new techniques are now available to isolate and remove the islet cells intact. In experimental diabetic animals certainly, injection of the islet cells has led to a cure or amelioration of the diabetic state. So far, many difficulties have to be overcome before islet cell transplants can be used in man. Nobody is quite sure what would happen if islet cells were transplanted into human subjects. They might be rapidly destroyed, they might proliferate or they might become malignant. At any rate, nobody is going to take risks in this respect, and here again much work has to be done before this could become a practical probability. The source of healthy islet cells could be obtained from the pancreas glands of stillborn babies born of healthy mothers. The pancreas gland of a new born baby contains a great number of islet cells, all of them capable of producing insulin.

5. STUDIES ON THE RETINA

As has been discussed, long-standing diabetes often leads to changes in the retina at the back of the eye and since these changes can lead to diminution in vision, great efforts have been made to discover the nature and cause of these changes. The retina can be compared to the film in a camera that records light images: it consists of light-sensitive nerve cells and fine blood vessels which course through it to supply the cells with oxygen and nourishment. When the retina is damaged in diabetes, inspection through the ophthalmoscope reveals changes in the calibre and shape of the blood vessels, and white areas of nerve cell damage. These changes have been observed in the retinae of animals rendered diabetic and, as in man, the duration of diabetes is the most important factor in inducing these changes. Thus four years of diabetes is necessary in the dog before retinal damage can be observed and at least six months in the rat. Dissection and microscopic examination of such retinae reveal significant weaknesses in the capillary walls. These tiny vessels show bulges known as microaneurysms and it seems likely that these fragile areas are liable to rupture and cause small haemorrhages. Examination under the electron microscope shows patchy thickening of the basement membrane, similar to that already mentioned in the islet cells and in the kidney glomeruli. The nerve cells of the retina may show areas of degeneration corresponding to the white areas seen through the ophthalmoscope. It is a matter for further study to determine whether these white exudates are due to toxic changes in the retina from improper nutriment or whether they result from damage to the capillaries supplying them. If the former supposition is true, it is important to study the metabolism of the nerve cells and much experimental work has been done on animal retinal tissue comparing normal with diabetic in respect of such biochemical parameters as glucous, fatty acids and mucopolysaccharides. In particular, comparative analysis of the basement membrane in diabetics and non-diabetics shows significant biochemical changes in the composition of this structure.

New techniques have been devised for the investigation of the retina in man. Fluorescein angiography involves the injection of fluorescein into a vein. Retinal photographs or cinephotography under ultraviolet light has made it possible to study the flow of fluorescein through the retinal vessels in great detail with elucidation of the nature of the abnormalities that occur in these vessel walls.

6. BABIES OF DIABETIC MOTHERS

Diabetes is known to exert a detrimental effect on the foetus (unborn baby). Many women who develop diabetes in later life have previously been delivered of large babies, weighing over 10 lb, perhaps twenty or thirty years before the onset of actual diabetes. Diabetic women who become pregnant also develop large babies, the increase in size and weight of the foetus usually occurring after the twenty-eighth week of pregnancy. These puzzling facts have stimulated a great deal of investigation. It seems unlikely that the raised blood sugar is the cause of these changes since they occur in women who have not yet developed diabetes and have normal blood sugars. The babies born to diabetic mothers tend to be overweight and plethoric but if they survive the first few days, their later development is normal. Of those who die, the pancreas gland shows a tremendous increase in the size and number of insulin-producing islet cells. Investigations into these problems have been pursued in different ways.

1. The possibility exists that the big babies are due to excessive production of growth hormone from the pituitary gland. It is known that growth hormone can induce diabetes, and excessive amounts would explain the increased size of the babies. But in fact, although some workers have demonstrated a raised level of growth hormone in some diabetic women during pregnancy, this finding does not always occur. Furthermore, excessive growth hormone leads to increased musculature and bone formation, whereas in these babies the increased size is due to fat.

2. The placenta, which nourishes the foetus in the womb, is usually increased in size during a diabetic pregnancy. The placenta is known to be a source of a number of hormones, some of which have been demonstrated in excess in diabetes. No convincing evidence exists that abnormal placental hormones are responsible for foetal changes.

3. The most plausible explanation of the increased size of the foetal islet cells is that excess maternal sugar enters the foetal circulation

and stimulates the foetal pancreas to produce more insulin. Investigations on newborn babies of diabetic mothers reveal that they have excess insulin and they are more capable of disposing of glucose than babies born of non-diabetic mothers. The main difficulty in accepting this theory has been stated, namely that women destined to develop diabetes often have large babies with large islet cells long before there is any detectable evidence of a raised blood sugar.

7. POPULATION STUDIES

The diagnosis of diabetes depends on the ability to dispose of a glucose load. In a suspected case, glucose is administered and the sugar in the blood measured at intervals. Normally the blood sugar should not exceed, say, 160 mg/100 ml and levels above this figure are defined as diabetic. Nevertheless, this level is an arbitrary one chosen merely for a convenient definition. Whereas there is general agreement that high blood sugars are a harmful abnormality associated with coronary thrombosis and other complications unless treated, we are less sure of the significance of levels of blood sugar only slightly elevated above what we define as normal. With this sort of problem in mind, studies of general populations have been undertaken, for example at Leicester and at Bedford, and analysis made of the findings, particularly of the borderline group who were neither obviously diabetic nor clearly normal. People in this group have been followed up for several years and the glucose tolerance tests repeated. Perhaps surprisingly, whereas some of those in this group developed diabetes over five years, the majority remained unchanged or even improved. Opportunity was also taken to see if tolbutamide, a sulphonylurea which lowers the blood sugar, would improve the health of those in this category by reducing the risk of coronary disease and allied complications. This work is proceeding, but so far no definite conclusion can be reached.

This chapter has set out to do no more than indicate some of the lines on which research is proceeding to elucidate the many unanswered problems in our understanding of diabetes.

INDEX